For Helmut

German edition:

Part 1:

Adieu colitis
Meine Wege aus der Krankheit
Wie ich durch Ernährungsumstellung gesund wurde

Part 2:

Darm über Kopf
Erfahrungsberichte
Vom erfolgreichen Kampf gegen unheilbare Krankheiten

3nd Edition 2019

© edition [zwischenräume] 14979 Großbeeren
Birkenstraße 12 www.vitale-landküche.de

Cover, typography and illustrations:

Michaela Barthel

www.barthel-art.de

ISBN 978-3-9815286-8-8

Michaela Barthel

Farewell Colitis

My journey out of my condition
or
How I became healthy by changing my diet

edition [zwischenräume]

2nd Edition – A few words before I begin

For seven years I suffered with ulcerative colitis, for seven years the condition defined my life and that of my family. I had to endure seven years of suffering before I was able to regain my old life through discipline and making changes to my diet and lifestyle. My incredibly supportive family was also instrumental in my success. I did not choose this illness; it was an unwelcome intruder. One that increasingly took decisions on the course that my daily life would take.

What is ulcerative colitis? It is a chronic inflammatory bowel condition which usually presents as periodic flare-ups and is accompanied by severe bleeding and pain. According to conventional medicine, it is a condition that cannot be cured.

So why have I written this book? After many years of living with this burdensome illness, I have found ways to escape my nightmare. Since this discovery, I have been able to live symptom-free and without the need for medication. For over two years now, I have had no symptoms of arthritis, even in my hands. As the years have gone by, I have become stricter and more experienced with my diet. I no longer want to imagine my life without wholefoods.

I am increasingly being asked for help from other people living with this condition who are also looking for an escape route. This prompted me to give presentations and offer cookery and baking courses, which I have been doing for a few years now. I have written about my experiences in this book. I would really like you to join me on my journey because I am convinced that much of the advice in this book can help other people suffering with ulcerative colitis. However, it must be borne in mind that everyone's journey to discover their own causes is a personal one and that you must be open to changing much about your existing lifestyle. Everyone's life and everyone's physical constitution is different. So my experiences are not necessarily going to be the same as yours. Moreover, the duration and severity of the illness are major factors. But I firmly believe that, at the very least, an improvement in the overall condition is achievable. The reason I believe this is because I have already met many people for whom it has also worked.

Why did I become ill? I have asked myself this time and time again. Why did I have to suffer in this way? There is a reason for everything. Why is it often so difficult to get the right diagnosis?
The causes of our symptoms have their roots in our pasts: in the lives we have led, our childhoods, our relationships with other people, how we live and work and how we are as individuals. A major factor here is that we no longer lead lives in tune with nature; one that involves natural nutrition, plenty of exercise and a healthy lifestyle. This is why this condition, like so many others, is one of the illnesses associated with the modern way of life. Our bodies repair themselves on a daily basis, often without us noticing. They send out clear cries for help in the form of pain. If we ignore these cries, at some point, our bodies will rebel and the damage can no longer be undone. We need to learn to listen and respond to what our bodies are telling us. It is possible to learn how to do this, but it can take a while, as I found out ...

My roots

I was born in 1960 and came from a typical East German family. My mother was a bookseller and my father held a doctorate in Economics. My parents worked all day long.
Before I came into this world, they had to cope with a particularly difficult period in their lives. My two-year old sister was often ill. This was a constant, daily struggle for my parents. At the same time, my father was convalescing from severe jaundice. My mother had just been discharged from a respiratory clinic having received prolonged treatment for pleurisy. Once discharged from the clinic, they were advised by the doctor to

travel to Thuringia for a holiday to recover. I was the result of their having spent more time with each other and their returning strength.

My mother had been unable to breastfeed me because she was having to take strong, long-term medication for her illness. Nevertheless, I was a healthy child. My brother was born two years later.

Daily life became much easier for my parents once they were able to swap our large, old, four-room, fifth-floor apartment with stove heating for a three-room, new build apartment with central heating. I still remember to this day how we children would help carry up the coal on Sundays during the winter. Even my little brother would trudge up the five staircases from the cellar to the top floor several times with a handful of coals. The compromise for district heating and mod cons however was a much smaller living space. 57-square metres meant that we had to share a small bedroom between the three of us.

Around the time that I went to school, my parents rented a small garden in the middle of the leafy Berlin district of Köpenick.

This garden was paradise for us. At the weekends, we would play in the sand, run through the woods and swim in every lake, or pull worms from the compost and try our luck at fishing. We would eat the produce from the garden without washing it.

Why am I mentioning this, you may wonder? Well, one possible cause for chronic inflammatory bowel diseases is thought to be that the stricter hygiene regimes in childhood these days mean that the immune system is less primed. So in my case, I've been able to rule this out as a possible cause for my condition.

My older sister was my role model as a child. She knew how to manage her siblings. At school she achieved very good results and was allowed to attend a special school from the third grade. Even though much was not easy for her, she always managed to make the best of things. She was popular wherever she went, always the first and always the best.

Back then, I felt that my younger brother – as the onlyboy –
was the golden child. He was of unshakeable health and a very
easy-to-care-for toddler. He quickly overtook me in size and
strength and was very assertive, so I am a middle child, a so-
called sandwich child, as psychologists say.

My favourite playmate was my sister of course, due to our close-
ness in age. She would often say to me, "Self-help helps yourself". The same applied when we played together. Almost all
the toys that we used in role plays with our dolls were our own
creations. All the accessories sold by the toy industry for the
likes of Barbie, etc., we would build, sew and create ourselves,
from dolls' school books to platform shoes, clothes and school
bags, right through to our very own dolls' houses.
These games allowed me to live out my imagination and creativity.
My sister was always amazed at me when I created things that
were important to our game but which she didn't have the time
to make. This taught me that being independent, working hard
and having imagination and perseverance were rewarded; I felt
happy and on an equal footing.
The relationship with my brother, however, was characterised
more by a competitive need for recognition from my parents.
At times of conflict especially, I often felt that my parents
wouldn't judge the situation fairly and that my younger brother
had the upper hand, and knew how to use it. This sometimes
made me feel like I wasn't loved or acknowledged enough.
In order to receive the same love and recognition from my parents as my siblings, I developed a lot of ambition in school and
in my hobbies. Among my lasting memories are being recognised for my ability to teach myself the guitar and making an
elaborate picture book of all the countries in the world for my
geography lesson. I drew maps that earned me lots of praise
from my favourite teacher and my classmates. Perhaps it was
when I was turning my many ideas into reality that I laid the
first foundation stone for over-stretching myself later on.
Today, I look back on my childhood and youth with great fond-
ness. I have particularly fond memories of the afternoons I spent

doing sports. Exercise and sport are second nature to me. That's why I tried out different disciplines. As I was a very good swimmer, I registered with a sports club and went training several times a week with friends. When I was swimming, I especially enjoyed how my body felt in the water, and I was happy doing it – even if some days my hair developed a greenish tinge. Being a child, I had no idea what chlorine was actually for.
I spent a lot of time reading from an early age. I was a real bookworm. To me, books were always synonymous with a magical world. I loved stories that allowed my imagination to run wild. They eased my soul, since good always triumphed. When I was reading, my parents really struggled to bring me back from my "dream world", and it would take me a while to get used to reality again.

For as long as I can remember I have had a great love of painting and drawing. It gave me great pleasure – and apparently I have quite a talent for it. I received admiration for my work, not only in my drawing class but also from friends, and especially from my father.
Because of this, my parents drew my attention to a newspaper article which mentioned a drawing and painting group in what was then the house of the painter, Otto Nagel. The free course was run by very well-known painters such as Konrad Knebel and Antje Fretwurst-Colberg and, in later years, by Christa and Lothar Böhme. I went there for many years with enthusiasm and success. Even as a child, my work was exhibited at regular amateur exhibitions in various galleries across East Berlin. I also became acquainted with various graphic design techniques here. Though I could never have imagined making painting my profession.

It was my love of books coupled with my creative talent that awakened my desire for a career in book design. Since I knew that study places were beyond rare and that the competition was extremely tough, I wanted to give myself the best start on the career ladder as I could. So, as well as the painting group, I attended an evening course in nature studies with the famous

Berlin graphic designers and artists, Wolfgang Leber and Wulf Sailer.

During my careers advice sessions, I learned that, in addition to talent, practical training in the graphic arts would also be beneficial if I wanted to obtain one of the coveted study places for typography. So I went on to complete an apprenticeship as a typesetter in lead typesetting. I learned the old and beautiful craft of the type case. For health and safety reasons, I had to drink a quarter of a litre of milk a day to prevent lead poisoning. Wearing gloves to reduce direct contact with the lead was not common practice and also impossible, since it would have been too difficult to grasp the tiny letters.

After successfully completing this training, I applied for my long-awaited typography degree and was accepted. I was thrilled to have passed all preliminary examinations and to have received one of only five available places. It was a dream come true for me. The school's objectives were based strongly on the Bauhaus movement and were very practical. The workshops and facilities were well-equipped in terms of space and resources. In addition to creativity, good organisational skills were particularly in demand, as it would be necessary to make a lot out of very little in a later career.

It was during my studies that my daughter Franziska was born. She was a very healthy child and a real ray of sunshine. Even though the stress was tremendous, I remember this time as being a very happy one. I was healthy and enjoyed motherhood and my young family.
After completing my studies, I was employed as a graduate, as was customary in East Germany, according to state-planned conventions. I really would have liked to have chosen a publisher that published children's books. But, as a young mother, the cards were stacked against me compared to male applicants, since in the East, I was also classed as a default risk.
In the years that followed, I was in great shape physically. Despite the many stresses, such as my job as a young professional,

the extensive expansion to an initially uninhabitable shop apartment in the Friedrichshain district, I didn't have any serious physical complaints.

My marriage to Helmut, the birth of my second daughter Josefine in 1987 and relocating our family to a new, airier apartment was the happiest time of my life. I derived great pleasure from my work; as their first graphic designer I had a lot of responsibility and success in the publishing house. My daily routine included – and still includes – doing regular sports and a lot of exercise in the fresh air.

1989 – Reunification

During the time of German reunification, a lot changed in our lives and professionally everything changed. Not only was the political and economic system in the former German Democratic Republic experiencing radical change, but so too was my entire field of work: typesetting technology.
The new technical marvel, the magical machine, now had a name: the Apple Macintosh. Desktop computers gained a foothold in the industry. All of a sudden, an incredible amount of things were possible. My job description as a graphic designer and typographer changed in just a few months through the use of computer technology. The many different professions that were previously instrumental in the production of books or magazines were reduced down to almost a single job! "Desktop publishing" was the new mot du jour. With a single computer, it was now possible to combine everything from editing to graphics and image processing into a complete layout in just a short space of time.
Up until this point in time, I had painstakingly pieced together the book title from individual letters or lines using a magnifying glass and images were laboriously processed in a photographic laboratory. These individual parts then had to be assembled in a complex and precise "handicraft work" to form a print template.

As a typographer, I was particularly impressed by the large number of fonts now readily available, the size of which I could change electronically and could immediately see a result on the screen. (What you see is what you get!). Also graphic shapes and illustrations could be designed freely on the computer and directly linked to the font. On the one hand, this was time-saving yet, on the other it had now taken over the work of numerous professionals!

Though, all these options could only be used if the company also had enough money to make the necessary investments. This wasn't clear-cut for the publisher for which I worked as a graphic designer. Nevertheless, I educated myself about these new technical possibilities at trade fairs and open day events. It was while doing this that I got an offer to visit an advertising agency in Wuppertal, which was looking for contacts with companies in East Germany.

It was at this time that my husband had also started a completely new job. He saw no future prospects in his role as a teacher of biology and chemistry, the need for science teachers had diminished; he decided to retrain in marketing. We travelled together for a week to Wuppertal and were able to extensively test the technical capabilities of Desktop Publishing on the Apple computers.

The openness and hospitality with which we were greeted there were remarkable. Even our hosts were just learning how to use this new DTP technology and our own solid, professional training made us an acknowledged partner.

As a result of this visit and after an initial training period, we received an offer to set up a subsidiary of the agency in Leipzig. We were overwhelmed by the opportunities and prospects and, after a few weeks of reflection, we decided to take the plunge. The decision was made all the easier due to there being little in the way of prospects for me at the publishing house.

However, taking this path created a challenge for our family life. We lived in Berlin and the work locations would be Leipzig and Wuppertal. School attendance and childcare had to be reorganised. Initially, Franziska moved in with my parents so that she wouldn't have to change primary school. Josefine spent the entire week with my brother-in-law's family near Leipzig and attended the local nursery with her cousin. Since we were working 16 to 18-hour days, our daughters lived most of the time with other families. After a long motorway journey, our family life was limited to the short weekend. I found this hugely stressful because even the children were not happy with this nomadic lifestyle. We lost out on that really important family time in the mornings and evenings, eating meals together, the chance to talk about and reflect on everything that had happened during the day. As parents, we could only give them limited love, warmth and security during this time.

Anyone who knows post-reunification Leipzig knows that there was a lack of affordable housing here. We finally gave up trying to change the situation and trying to find a place to live in Leipzig after months of unsuccessfully searching. It was clear to us that we didn't want to live like this anymore. We were encouraged in our decision after the agency's parent company, a large Apple dealer, wanted to close the Leipzig location since the economic boom expected in the East was a long time coming.

The path to independence

Unemployment was not a consideration for us, especially since we were offered a large contract almost at the same time. We therefore thought about starting our own business. We were attracted by the opportunity to set up our own company and make independent decisions. We had already experienced how an agency worked. We were now convinced that our professional training provided us with a good basis. The rest we would have to learn. (That's how you see it when you're young, the working hours for "learning by doing" turned some nights into days). But the best thing about this attitude was that the family could finally be together again!

Of course, we also had lots of concerns. We were a young family with responsibility for four children since Oliver and Sascha, Helmut's children, were also part of the family, mostly at the weekends. The order situation was still very manageable. Loans were out of the question due to a lack of collateral. At that time there were no state-sponsorship programmes for start-ups. We just had us, our knowledge and our enthusiasm.

We therefore initially set up our company in our four-room apartment. The children now had to share the smallest bedroom. The former children's bedroom became the office. At the same time, we were looking for an affordable solution which would enable us to live and work under the same roof or as close as possible to our home. The commercial property situation in Berlin in the period following reunification wasn't exactly rosy, which is why our search for a property ended up taking us more than a year. The offers were well above our budget or failed due to the lack of collateral that young entrepreneurs from the East simply didn't have.

We finally struck it lucky in Brandenburg with a newly built, end terrace in a small town in the affluent suburbs. There was enough space for both the family and the company here. The basement office even had a separate entrance. The new house was a dream come true for the children because they each had their own bedroom with a balcony and a view of the garden. We were very happy and loved living and working in the countryside. The girls quickly got used the new surroundings and made new friends. Franziska went to school in the village, which wasn't too far at all.

Changing our diet

An important – but barely noted – change in daily life over these last few years has been our diet. The constant commute between the place where we worked and where we lived and time pressures led to food taking a back seat, apart from at the weekends. We made full use of the wide variety of sweets, processed foods and coffee that was now available to us in order to overcome hunger, stress and tiredness.

Even after our move, this did not change significantly. As well as bread, potatoes, pasta and frozen products, our staple diet naturally consisted of tinned foods, baked goods and foods which have a long shelf-life and are handy for transporting, such as milk or juices in Tetra-Paks. At that time, we didn't have a supermarket where we lived. In addition, we tried many things from the wide range of foods, including processed products such as cakes and pizzas and yoghurt with fruit preparations.

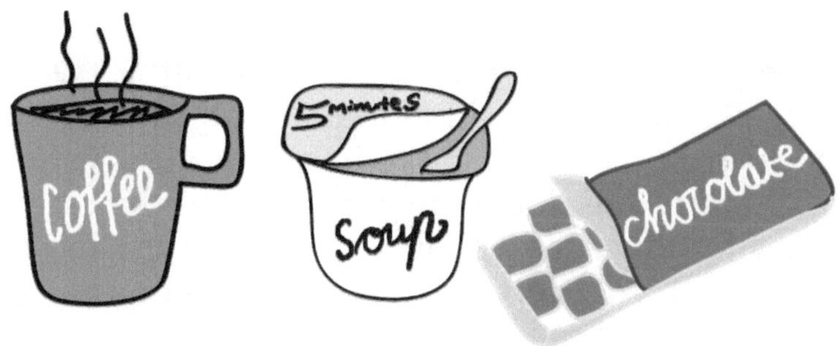

All this was always available. The appeal of the huge consumer choice seduced us, too. Without doubt, somewhere in the subconscious, the experiences of having such shortages in East Germany will have played their part. We were also doing the advertising for many products, and had to try out for ourselves whether they really were as great as they were being presented.

Independence

The early years, in particular, were one continuous frenzy. The endless stream of new technical possibilities captivated me every day.
Our motto during this period was "learning by doing". We learnt how to use the technological possibilities and with every success, our expectations in terms of outcomes and those of our customers increased. Image editing and montage were com-

pletely new worlds, even if the programs were still simple compared to today's possibilities. Drawing programs made it possible to display graphics, logos and illustrations with a completely new variety and complexity.

The snag was getting things from screen to paper. Much of what was possible on the computer could only be captured on the printing plate and then printed in the desired quality with great difficulty. The technology providers and service providers were also in the process of learning. This took time and sometimes led to situations that reached the limits of their capabilities. In the background there was always the pressure to achieve economic success.

Nevertheless, during these years I felt very healthy. I was always fit and active. Now and again I would get a slight pain in my hip joint which would cause me to hobble around for days.

I assumed that this was due to my prolonged, sedentary job, because sitting for long periods puts a strain on the joints, especially the hips. I was certainly not doing enough sporting activities but I had no time for that.

However, the pain gradually increased. I ignored it due to time constraints. It actually got to the point where I could completely block it out. I would then only feel the pain again when it became stronger or when my stress eased.

The symptoms usually appeared suddenly and unexpectedly; it felt like a stabbing pain in the right hip. I then had to stay standing up and couldn't move. I shifted my weight to my pain-free joint to relieve the burden on the other one. Swinging my leg slowly increased the range of movement. Eventually, I was able to sit down again. These moments disrupted my tightly organised daily routine and I was trapped in my own body because I was unable to achieve anything.

Exercise has always been so important to me because it makes me feel good. I used to be sporty, so I assumed I always would be. I didn't want to accept any change as far as this was concerned. My body was forcing me to slow down, but I ignored it. I simply could not allow myself to be hindered, no matter what.

At that time, I had nobody to talk to about my symptoms. Back then, my friends, like us, were going through huge professional changes. Many had left the city and moved with their families to the western states. We had plenty of other topics of conversation to discuss for the few hours that we visited each other or talked on the phone. I didn't want to burden these conversations with talk of "health" or "illness". They knew that we worked a lot but my slowly emerging health problems were a taboo topic. I had avoided talking about them, the subject wasn't particularly attractive and it wasn't important enough to me. I didn't even go to see the doctor in the beginning.

After being self-employed for about five years, I sat down for the first time and thought about how much sport I was still doing – at 34 years of age. I regularly went swimming as a child and a young girl. I loved sport in school, especially gymnastics and floor exercises as well as track-and-field athletics and long-distance running. I had also regularly engaged in sport, even when my daughter, Franziska was born. Things had been very different since we started our own business: I wasn't doing sport anymore, I was travelling everywhere by car, sitting down the entire day, usually spending 12 to 16 hours at the computer, even at the weekend. I would take the children (in the car) each week to equestrian vaulting and the small garden at the terrace house was not suitable for the weekly turning over of the soil. I was well aware of the problem but I was lacking the initiative to change it.

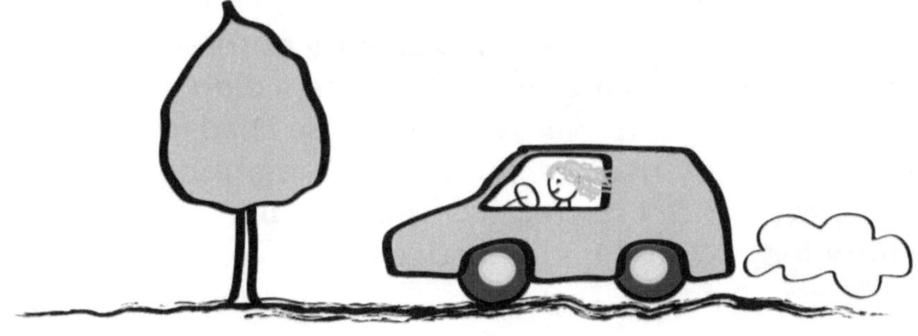

The illness years

1997

Repression

The illness started in the spring. When I first saw blood in my stools, I was shocked. I don't need a doctor, I thought. I was sure this apparition would disappear as quickly as a nosebleed does. Using this as a comparison, I managed to calm myself down. However, after a few days, the bleeding returned. I told myself that if it got worse, I would go to the doctor. The doctor would find out what the problem is and would help me.
For a long time I suppressed the fear when the blood returned. If I didn't see any blood, that was one more reason to ignore any negativity. Just finish this job, meet the deadlines, and when everything is done, I'll take care of it.

When a friend asks what a self-employed person does, there is often the flippant explanation: well, they're employed by them-selves, of course. And that's exactly how I saw my life. Without me, nothing would happen and if I did nothing, I wouldn't earn any money. In a manner of speaking, this was true but also false. As such I would often put myself under great pressure at work. The results were tension in the neck and shoulder muscles and this would in turn give me a headache. To combat this I drank coffee. Four to five cups a day was quite normal at that time. I never felt great drinking so much coffee. I didn't like the smell it left on my body afterwards. But because I had low blood pressure I particularly needed coffee in the morning. It had been this way ever since I started working. If I didn't drink coffee in the morning, I would get a headache and wouldn't be able to shake it off all day.

I would then feel noticeably worse in the meantime. Eventually, I had to think about what I was going to do about it.
What kind of doctor do you go to when your bowel is bleeding? I didn't have a clue. I had absolutely no idea who could help me. What happens during the examination? What will the doctors do to me to find out the cause of what is making my bowel bleed? Who could I confide in? In addition, I didn't know any doctors in the village, as we had only lived here for a few years. That was another welcome reason for me to push this unpleasantness away from me.

My body –
an indestructible workhorse?

A few days without symptoms always gave me the hope that this was all only temporary. I would then assume that it would regulate itself because I thought of my body as an indestructible workhorse.
The disease, however, did not feel that I was taking it seriously. It wanted its voice to be heard and therefore spread further, without asking my permission. Each time I deteriorated, my fear grew. But instead of going to the doctor, I was afraid of going to the toilet.
I was now seeing blood on regular occasions. I then started experiencing diarrhoea and pain. What did I know of illness and disease in my mid-30s?
It was August when I finally plucked up the courage to speak to my husband about my symptoms. I hadn't wanted to worry him and until that moment had said nothing. Helmut was baffled as to why I hadn't told him and, at the fact that I STILL HADN'T been to the doctor. Of course, he was right and he was extremely concerned about my well-being. Later, I often asked myself why I had neglected my health and what other way there could have been. The most important reason that kept

coming to mind was that I hadn't wanted to jeopardise the development of our business. And of course, I didn't want to leave my husband high and dry with lots of projects to do. I enjoyed my work, it was varied and demanding, I couldn't just stop. I was a workaholic.

Our way of working was based on the fact that we complemented each other perfectly. Everyone did what they were best at. Helmut's areas of responsibility were marketing consultancy, public relations and developing advertising strategies, personnel issues and technology. From this, I developed the communication concept, created the design, the presentation and the individual advertising media.
Initially, book designs and technical illustrations played the main role, but these were increasingly supplemented by overall concepts for garden centres and DIY stores. The work pressure increased significantly. By spring we had taken on a new employee to take the load of the many administrative office duties from our shoulders. Then we sought further help in the area of image processing and archiving of the ever increasing number of productions. We received a huge number of applications from candidates; generally people retraining or those seeking a lateral career move since this job description had only existed for a year.
Before long, we had to acknowledge that a lengthy learning period would be required for these employees. That prompted us to consider setting up our own apprenticeship training scheme. We wanted to have qualified junior staff first-hand, so to speak. More than 100 applications for two trainee places proved that there was great interest in this domain. The choice was equally time-consuming. Of course, it was clear to us that apprenticeship training meant increased effort to start with. In addition to my own work, it was my job to train the young employees. It all worked out in the end and our trainees did very well.

In November, almost nine months after the noticing the first signs, I was finally ready and wanted to confide in my female gynaecologist. She was the doctor that I hadn't wanted to change after we moved to Brandenburg because she had known me for a long time and I had only ever had positive experiences with her up until then. I was now experiencing regular bleeding, pain and anxiety due to diarrhoea, and constant weakness, fatigue and exhaustion deprived me of more of my strength every day.

The diagnosis

At the end of November 1997, I had the appointment with my gynaecologist. She immediately diagnosed ulcerative colitis. My symptoms now had a name. I had never heard of this condition before and so I couldn't really imagine what it might be. The findings were: *(1. chronically-recurring proctitis, grade III with erosions, ... 2. chronically-recurring proctitis, grade II-III with micro-haemorrhages. Swelling ... at the level of 10 cm.)*

The laboratories only confirmed the diagnosis. *(Chron. recurr. proct. grade III with erosions, ulcerations, pseudopolypoid hyperplasia, crypts ... no evidence of malignancy. The findings are consistent with ulcerative colitis).* Because I couldn't imagine exactly what this meant, the diagnosis was shocking for me. "The causes are not known", I learned from my doctor. "The condition has been quite rare so far, but has become more common in recent years. For a long time, psychological stress was assumed to be the cause, but this has now been dismissed, since these stresses were usually linked to living with the disease itself. But stress could still have played an important role," she explained to me. She also mentioned that people who were not breastfed as babies were more likely to be affected by this disease, and that there could be a hereditary link. "Do you have this condition in the family?", she asked. "No, I've got a big family but I don't know of anyone in my family with this."
"What are the possibilities of curing it?", I asked.
"Well, there's a lot that can be done, there are some new drugs

on the market. Previously, it was much more difficult...", she prescribed me some suppositories. I trusted my doctor. I knew that she had sufficient experience.

I drove home, feeling calm and hopeful. If only I'd gone there sooner, it would have saved me so much pain and stress!
I handed the prescription in at the pharmacy and collected the medication the very next day. It was as simple as that. A few days later and the bleeding stopped completely. For me, back then, a visit to the doctor meant that I was as good as cured.
I was so relieved when I noticed that after a few days the suppositories were clearly working! It was a great feeling. I was going to be alright! After just a few days, my symptoms had disappeared and I was feeling well. I had renewed optimism, my head was clearer again. I was keen to tackle the new projects that were lying on my desk, even though I couldn't yet muster up the strength that I would have otherwise been able to draw on. But that would return, of course. I was filled with hope!
The basement office was too small for four employees, especially since we planned to add two more employees to the fold in the near future. So we began searching for suitable premises and struck lucky after just a few weeks. We found an attractive solution in an industrial park ten kilometres away: 170 square metres, seven rooms, light, spacious and available immediately. We were thrilled that the move could take place soon, before the year was out.

At this time, I realised that my prescribed medicine ONLY WORKED FOR A FEW WEEKS. The illness had obviously not been defeated because my intestinal bleeding started again. I was shocked by this. I couldn't understand why the medication intended for this condition had not helped. It seemed worse than I'd feared. I was going to have to take this illness more seriously, I thought. I called my doctor and we discussed that we would wait until the end of the year, when things would be calmer, and we would arrange another appointment for January. We had the 1997 Christmas holidays off. Three days dedicated to the family. Time for a cosy Christmas, some peace, playing with the children, enjoying and eating well. I longed for peace, for long winter walks. I had forgotten what time-out was, what a holiday was. However, the illness didn't improve despite this. The symptoms continued to increase.

23

Medication costs in 1997: 12.69 Euro

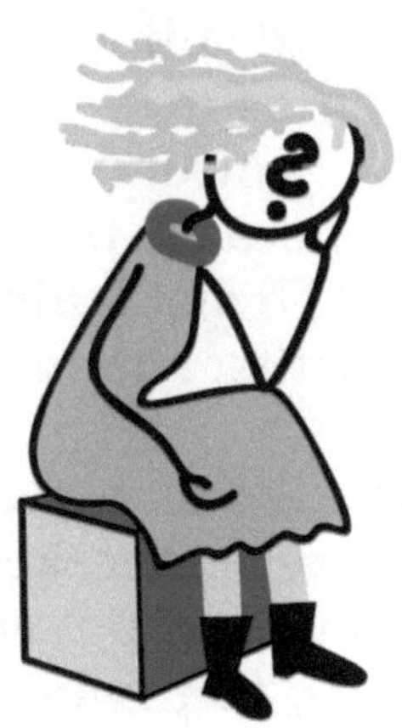

1998

New hope

I went back to see my doctor at the start of January. "The findings are consistent with moderate florid colitis. Compared to the previous examination, there is a marked improvement." However, my doctor was not happy with this and, of course, neither was I, although I was somewhat better than before my first visit to the doctor. I was now given a new medication instead of the suppositories, since the effect of these was not sufficient. Salofalk 500, an anti-inflammatory, was the new drug. One tablet contains 500 mg of mesalazine (5-aminosalicylic acid) as its active ingredient. I was given a large white tub containing 300 tablets: I had to take 3 of these tablets daily.

I wanted to know more about this condition from my doctor because an improvement, albeit in small steps, was clearly possible. So I asked her how I could help the healing process, what I should eat and what I should avoid. To me it was obvious that the diarrhoea and intestinal problems had to be linked to nutrition. But she explained to me that this condition was rarely affected by food. It would be important for me to eat a varied diet. I was advised to eat meals, little and often, all well cooked or steamed, and with little fried fat. I should avoid coffee and alcohol, but that was a given. I had already reduced my coffee intake because it stimulated the urge to pass a bowel movement. But I didn't want to cut it out entirely because of my headaches. I would only have to consume this bland diet during the acute inflammatory phase. She asked me whether I had any unusual eating habits.

I recited a list of what our family mealtimes consisted of: brown bread, white bread, bread rolls, sometimes cakes, pancakes, sponge cakes or home-made cakes. At lunchtimes, we'd have pasta, rice, potatoes, mash or roasted. Schnitzel, fish fingers, goulash, quark, cheese and eggs all regularly appeared on the table. Frozen pizzas were particularly popular with the children. It was their tastes that decided which brands made it into the shopping trolley.

Of course, we also had fruit, vegetables and salads in our daily diets. Quark dishes with fresh or preserved fruit were home-made, for example, with blackcurrants. However, yoghurt from the supermarket has always been a competitor because of the power of advertising and the fact that it's so readily available. Josefine loved the mini fruit yoghurts in particular. I usually cooked lunch myself. In doing so, I would also sometimes use processed foods as part of the ingredients, for example, gratin topping out of a packet.

From time to time, we also tried ready meals from the freezer, for example stir-fry vegetables or Chinese noodles. But we soon stopped that since Helmut, who never had any problems, repeatedly noticed that after eating these, his arms and the skin on his face would itch. I noticed a similar feeling when I ate ice cream from a street vendor. I would often get a numb feeling in my mouth afterwards.

Eating a varied diet was and is important to me, so I pay a lot of attention to it. In my opinion, I was doing everything right. This was the view of my doctor, too.

Even though she confirmed the fact that I was eating a good diet, I started to mull over what influence individual foods could be having on the course of the disease. I knew from my child-hood that puréed carrot or grated apple relieved stomach pain and helped to combat diarrhoea. Were there ingredients within my diet that could be responsible for this inflammation? The new medication was working well and I slowly began to feel better over the next few weeks. I had renewed hope and en-joyed this period of improvement.

In March, we came down with a severe flu-like infection, which we brought back with us from the CeBIT trade fair. The infec-tion was treated with the antibiotic Citromax. It was very pow-erful. Once over the infection, the colitis took a little break. I was able to briefly catch my breath and stabilise myself, but at the beginning of April, it came back with renewed vigour.

I had always felt that stress exacerbated the flare-ups and possibly even triggered them. I accepted that, for me, stress increased the activity of the disease. However I still had to perform equally well on a daily basis with a weakened body. But to what extent is stress a trigger for colitis? Is there any knowledge, any research? Why has it not been investigated? These were questions I often asked myself.
My body yearned for rest, for a break. I could feel it. But to be out of work for weeks or months, to leave the stress behind for once, how would that work?

Problems again

Then came another problem in the form of our new office. I now had a commute which I often couldn't cope with. Recurring, painful diarrhoea, which I was increasingly unable to control, was an obstacle to leaving the house. I had my own office, of course, which helped with these symptoms. But the long way to the toilet was problematic; I had to pass through all the other employees' offices then through two heavy doors and then I was met with a very long corridor! Fortunately, most of the office spaces were not rented. But the journey there was like running the gauntlet for me because I had no control over the diarrhoea and painful cramps as well as the gas which increasingly built up in my intestines due to the inflammation. My stomach would rumble loudly, it bubbled, and then my bowels would, very painfully, empty bloody stools and gas, which fizzled uncontrollably out of me.

Since we were also working for retailers, deadlines were crucial. The production of catalogues and inserts is planned ahead of time for the entire year with accompanying deadlines. Our advertising flyers have to be with the daily newspapers by a fixed date. There is no leeway in terms of time.
During the periods when I had flare-ups, I would try to manage my daily tasks. I would arrive late to the office and stay there

into the night. I hoped the better organised I was with my jobs, the quicker they would be done.

Often, however, things turned out very differently. Sometimes there would be technical issues, sometimes staff would be off work due to illness and I had to find a solution for the increased workload. Approaching final deadlines, this would lead to increased work pressure which then, instead of breathing a sigh of relief once the work was complete, caused me to have migraines.

New symptoms

My hands had been aching for several weeks. Typing on the keyboard was becoming harder every day. All my fingers, especially my index finger, would send out a constant throbbing pain and would swell. My joints were always very sensitive to pressure and my hands were always cold as ice. It was becoming increasingly impossible to type using all ten fingers. The smallest of movements caused me pain. I could only use my middle finger to type and that took much more time.

I wanted to do something to help my hands and so I looked for my fine, warm angora gloves, cut all ten fingertips off and crocheted around them so that the stitches didn't come undone. I hoped that the heat would make the pain more bearable but that didn't happen. The cause was therefore not the cold. What was it then? Something else I had to go and speak to my doctor about!

When I wasn't feeling well, I was very fretful and could only think of myself. I spent a lot of time visiting the toilet and the pain often completely exhausted me. I had simply blanked out many things, including family life. I was barely there for the children. Helmut had to respond daily to my changing condition. That demanded a lot of him. Especially when there were customer appointments or meetings in the offing, or when the trainees had a training session. If he saw that I was not in my room, he knew that I was not available. He reorganised or undertook any pending tasks without dispute or asking questions and all in addition to his own ever-increasing workload. Since I could no longer do my work during the day, I usually worked late into the night. When it was quieter in the office and the telephone had stopped ringing, I could relax and be myself more. I often felt better in the evenings.

I had severe hair loss for several weeks. Could this be linked to the new Salofalk medication? It was getting worse by the day. I have very long, thick hair.
The hairbrush was constantly full and long hair could be found all over my jacket, shoulders and the back of my chair. If anybody plucked the hair from my jacket or drew my attention to it while we were having a conversation, I would feel very embarrassed. It reminded me of my illness, of my "frailty" – even though I was blanking out the problem itself.
Hiding the illness and its limitations became more and more important to me; these were brief moments of relaxation for me. Far too rarely have I taken the time to relax in recent years. Now, I had started to enjoy these short moments: when I was walking in the countryside or spending time with the family and when I was just feeling well. When I did rest, the pain would subside, then I could switch off and felt almost normal and not hounded by my condition. I wanted to escape, run away from the illness. I struggled to accept the fact that I had to ask the illness for every little thing.

My GP examined me for thyroid dysfunction because of the hair loss. But to no avail. Added to this, diffuse alopecia (scalp eczema) started to spread over my head. My scalp became encrusted, weepy, tight and itchy. My dermatologist didn't really know much about my underlying condition or the medication I was taking. I had to explain it all to her and, as a precaution, I took the medication packaging leaflet along with me. I always read this through. I find it really confusing to read that the side effects include diarrhoea or joint problems. I wondered why I had even been prescribed this medication if this is the case. If I speak to my doctors about this, they will say that the medication is currently the best on the market and that the side effects are extremely rare.

Of course, I could always ask another doctor or pharmacist but would another doctor or pharmacist give me the same information? I was often not so sure about this but I didn't know what alternatives or similar medications were available.

I had now been prescribed Alpicort by the dermatologist and I also had to use oil packs to relieve my scalp and calm the weeping eczema.

I'm afraid

Besides the pain, the urgency to move my bowels was my greatest burden. It was the inability to hold it as soon as the urge to go to the toilet began. The rule was that if I didn't manage to hold it in, it would end up in my underwear. I was in a constant state of fear. The bowel movement starts spontaneously and with great pain. Once the pain gave its signal, it was already too late. It rarely forewarned me. It was involuntary, I had no control over it. Any desire to do so was quashed by the pain. What then followed, I would then experience with full consciousness, and I would be helplessly at the mercy of the situation because my intestines were not playing along; and so would anyone else around at the time.

Despite my handicap, during these phases, I tried to contribute every day by doing simple tasks and errands. But time and time again it went wrong, I found it all very depressing! In these situations I felt helpless, like a little child. It was usually Helmut who saved the day. He came to my aid or got me a change of clothes. Afterwards, I would often just cry. I felt that I became emotionally more unstable from time to time and repeatedly decided not to be so vulnerable, not to cry and to simply put behind me what had happened and look forward. I could always rely on Helmut, he managed to relax everything with just simple words. He radiated calmness or took me in his arms to comfort me.

My biggest stress was in the mornings. Barely any days started out relaxed anymore. Constant painful toilet visits – four to six times in the morning – were normal, then the intervals between visits would get longer and towards midday, everything would have calmed down. The burning and cramps diminished. I would use those breaks in between to get my strength back, I would lie exhausted on the bed and try to warm up my tortured and freezing body.

But the problems would reignite as soon as I wanted to leave the house. I would then no longer feel safe, my body took it as a new threat and reacted accordingly.

Doing those completely normal, everyday things such as visiting the towns or markets became increasingly impossible for me because there were rarely any toilets. You're not welcome in restaurants if you are not a guest. And public buildings are also difficult. If you go into one, the toilets are often difficult to find or are locked. In shopping centres, the toilets are usually located centrally. The route to which is through a maze of shops. All of which is just too far! Department stores often have toilets on the top floor and only supermarkets of a certain size have facilities. Public transport or train stations are impossible – everything is central. This is complicated by the fact that deadlines such as train departure times are an added pressure that the mind just can't cope with. Train station toilets are often overcrowded and difficult to find.

Walks are only possible if there is no chance of bumping in to anybody, a city park rarely has accessible toilets. And if it does, they tend to be locked, with the opening times kindly written on the door.

My fear and anxiety around leaving the house would rise further due to these everyday experiences. Contact with colleagues, friends, acquaintances, neighbours? – Not a chance, this became less and less.

Another two examples:
How do I shop in a supermarket?
A shopping trip to the supermarket had to be carefully planned. I couldn't simply go shopping, that was out of the question. It meant that I couldn't eat anything two hours beforehand. It was also important for me to know exactly where the toilets were located in the supermarket. At the supermarket, where we often go, I know exactly where they are. Right next to the entrance. In practical terms, going shopping for me means that all the way round the supermarket, I have to keep the shortest route to the toilet in the back of my mind. I arrange the route I take around the store according to these criteria. Shopping now takes much longer but this is the only way I can feel reasonably safe. The biggest obstacle to a successful shopping trip is the checkout, the conveyor belt. It's not possible to just run from here. My tactic is to not put my shopping on the conveyor belt until I feel safe. But there are times when I misjudge the situation and I take all my shopping off the conveyor belt and bundle it back into my trolley in a panic because I have to get to the toilet as a matter of urgency.

It would be really helpful if there were a special checkout, for example, at the information point in the foyer. In all fairness, I must admit that I have never asked anyone for this solution. I don't want to out myself as a UC patient and have to explain everything.

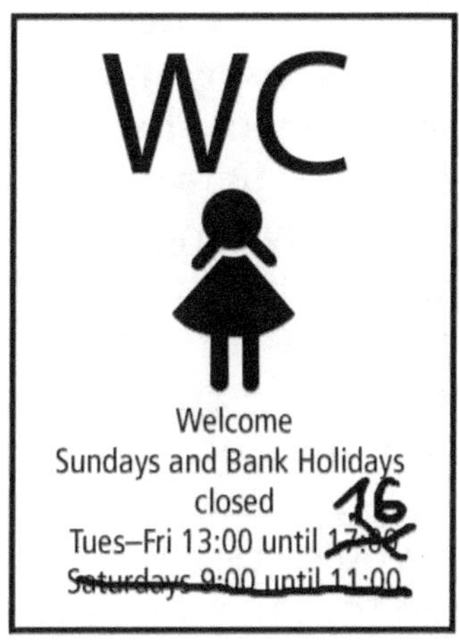

After leaving the checkout area, I then have to be sure that, in the event of a problem, my full trolley is not left unattended. This works really well in my supermarket because the friendly ladies at the counter in the foyer area always look after my shopping for me. I'm so grateful for that!
Close to where I live, there are now supermarkets within walking distance. These don't have toilets. I therefore have to drive the 200 meters to go shopping. Here I simply leave my full trolley by the shelves in an emergency, leave the supermarket and drive back home. When I come back, I often find that my trolley is still there.

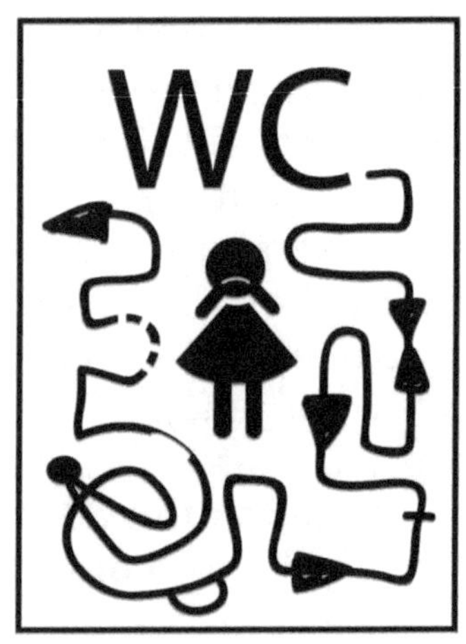

How do I go on business trips?
Of the few times that I can still remember and that I have gone alone, the following sticks in my mind: business trips always have to be meticulously planned. The most important thing was not to eat anything the night before; the second was to get up very early and to not eat anything early on and give the gut enough time to prepare for the day ahead. The third thing was to do everything calmly and with the necessary time buffer. Of course, this also included setting off in good time!
My aim was to get to the first service station in a relaxed state. Shortly before the first leg of the journey, that all-too-familiar burning and bubbling would start in my tummy. That was a bad sign. My hope was then to find a parking space in the immedi-

ate vicinity of the toilets. Unfortunately there were only disabled parking spaces near to the toilets and almost all other spaces were occupied! I wasn't brave enough to park in a disabled space because I was not considered disabled and therefore wasn't allowed to park there. I looked for another space but it was clear that I wasn't going to make it. It was now just a matter of the rectifying the consequences of those few minutes. As always, it was very depressing and it did little for my feeling of self-worth.

At the next service station, I drove slowly, I listened to myself. I was ok. I drove past and reached my appointment. I also had to go to the toilet several times during the meeting. My customer tolerated these interruptions and didn't ask any questions. Maybe this was because we had known each other for a long time. At a first meeting that undoubtedly would not have been possible. I took my time on the return journey. The relief at arriving home without having had any issues was immense and I felt so proud that I had done it! Later, I was helped out in these situations by a Euro-WC key. You can get the key from CBF-Darmstadt e.V. or from the DCCV in Germany. To apply for one, you need a doctor's certificate. Unfortunately, the key does not entitle you to park in disabled parking spaces. Of course, that would be even better and would not only have helped me in this particular situation.

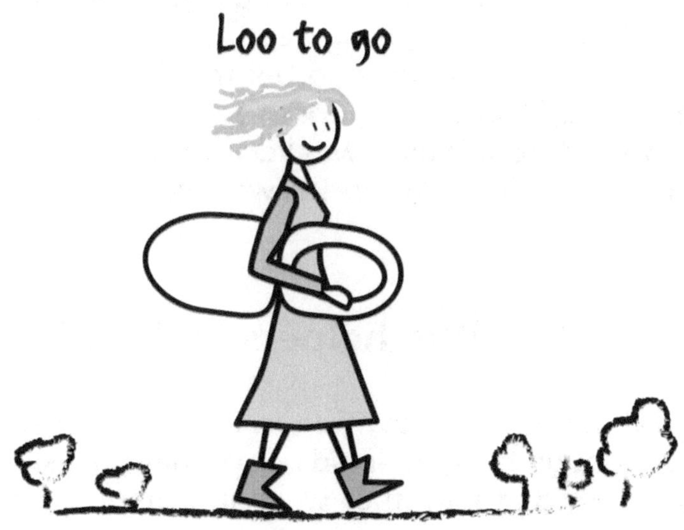

Over the summer I had a small period of remission, which meant that the illness was taking a bit of a rest. The order situation and the office organisation allowed us to take a three-week holiday. The destination of our trip was Brittany with a stopover in Paris. This trip was a dream come true for both the children and us. The children wanted to go to Disneyland and we wanted to enjoy the City of Love. In contrast, Brittany was a scenic discovery. My most vivid memories include the impressive Atlantic coast and a beautiful Breton wedding that we were able to witness. Our holiday home lay right on an estuary and had a mesmerising view. The pace of life was clearly French. This also included the enjoyment of home-made dishes made from freshly caught fish and local vegetables.

A holiday apartment with a second toilet was the right decision for this holiday. I had the rest that I needed and the rest of the family didn't have to queue for the toilet. After all, we were on holiday, and we didn't want any unnecessary frustration.

Unfortunately at the end of the summer, immediately after the holiday, this relative rest period came to an end.

A new, more severe flare-up of the disease began at the end of August:

"Florid ulcerative colitis, chronic recurrent grade III proctitis" was diagnosed. Severe joint pains in the hips started again. I found walking very difficult most days; I used tables, walls and railings to help me move around and often had to stop because I was incapable of moving at all.

The pain in my hands also became worse. I wrapped angora knitted cuffs around my wrists although these didn't have any positive effects. Typing was very difficult, my hands were bent and really stiff and my wrists were severely swollen.

Little helpers in the office

Our children had grown up in the 90s with Apple computers. Even though the games did not yet have the same graphic quality as they do today, they were an experience of a new kind. In our work, they were particularly interested in the ability to manipulate images as well as the drawing and graphics programs. They also learnt how to touch-type with ten fingers. And as is customary in a family business, the time came at some point when the children helped out in the business. We didn't have to push them since the job offered too many attractions.

Our daughter, Franziska was already 17 and willingly helped out in the office. She was interested in everything we were working on. She found it easy to grasp tasks and solve problems. She supported us with text entry, image processing or cartography.
Josefine was also busy practising on the keyboard with her ten little fingers; she was now 11 years old.
The children could of course use the skills they learnt in the office in their school work. Both have experimented and learned a lot when designing the covers of their exercise books or doing their homework. They were more than entitled to be proud of the results. Their excellent computer and typing skills would be useful to them in later life, not just in their ICT lessons.
If the children helped us in the office, they were able to increase their pocket money or amass working hours to finance their driving lessons, for example. Through this, they learnt from an early age that to earn money, you have to work hard.
When I see how well they are doing today in their professions and how independent they are in their lives, I'm so glad we involved them in the business. But of course it was also just so nice to have them with us in these moments.

At the rheumatologist's

Due to the increasing pain I was experiencing, my doctor recommended that I visit a rheumatologist and transferred me to the Charité University Hospital in Berlin. She wanted to get the advice of a specialist to ensure that everything was clear.
First, my wrists were x-rayed then my hip joints and an auto-an-

tibody and immune screening were conducted given the suspected diagnosis of arthritis with UC. Arthritis can occur with ulcerative colitis as a concomitant disease, she had already told me this. The doctor explained to me that because both diseases were autoimmune conditions, a common cause was to be assumed. The rheumatism can therefore be treated with the same active ingredient as that used in acute bouts of ulcerative colitis. That made me feel better because I was relying on the fact that I wouldn't have to take another form of medication because the burden of the side effects was adding to the burden of the illness.

The rheumatologist recommended that I increase the Salofalk to 3x2 tablets. In addition to the Salofalk, I was to use Colifoam rectal foam to suppress this flare-up with hydrocortisone more quickly and more effectively. This doctor also advised me to regularly take vitamin E; he said that it had always been a good support to him in times of stress.

The amount of medication I was taking increased with each new flare-up. It was never less medication, always more. This caused me increasing concern because this meant that the side effects also increased. I also had the feeling that with the increasing dosage of medication, my body would continue to get weaker and that I would have less and less energy for my daily work.

Over the next few days, a bacterial infection took a hold of my face and my mouth. The right side of my face was initially just red and tight. Then the skin started to split in different places, fluid oozed out and crusted over. My skin was flaky. The affected areas grew larger by the day and soon spread from my mouth across my right eye so much that I had to carefully dab it with a lime blossom teabag in the mornings just to be able to open it a little. I also suffered with conjunctivitis. Changes in the atmosphere, heat, cold, draughts and dry central heating were pure stress for my skin. The eczema also spread inside my mouth, this was extremely dry, tight and itchy. My lips were numb and chapped, I could only speak without moving my lips. I couldn't see properly, couldn't eat and couldn't communicate very well. Facial expressions were a strain – I couldn't even laugh. I felt wretched. A port wine stain of around 10 centimetres in diameter was now glowing on the right side of my neck. There were no signs that it would improve by itself; I had to go back to the doctor again.

I went to the dermatologist. It didn't matter what she said to me, what she did to me, what she prescribed me, so long as it would help! The symptoms were treated with Sobelin 300N, which I had to apply every hour. On the package insert, I later read that this active ingredient should be used with extreme care in patients with gastrointestinal conditions.

Difficult visits to the doctor

When I go to see the doctor, it is important for me to understand why the doctor is prescribing me something and what the side effects may be. Only then am I able to rank this drug amongst the multitude of drugs I am taking and give the appropriate feedback. Unfortunately, however, these side effects often occur before the next appointment date. Since appointments in between are often not available, I took myself off to see the dermatologist to try to get some relief for my symptoms. My knowledge of the medication and the side effects was vital for the doctor to be able to help me.

However, I often felt overwhelmed with this task, especially since I was never sure that I had described everything correctly and set the right focus. I often fear mentioning EVERY new problem because I don't want to receive LOTS OF new drugs. So, it is difficult to guess the effects of each individual medication and impossible to clearly determine which side effects are attributed to which drug. I was frequently under the impression that my doctor didn't know what to do when I presented myself before her with new symptoms and the packaging inserts. Undoubtedly the situation at that time was also to blame. Polyclinics no longer existed and communication between doctors, in particular between Brandenburg and Berlin was still very much in need of improvement.

Why is it that a doctor is only responsible for a certain area of the body? I was the "informant" between them. I often felt like I was stuck between two places, or like I was between the individual parts of my body. I became aware that not one of the doctors had looked for the causes of the new symptoms – maybe there was and is an alternative to the medication which had caused the side effects? It was always a matter of prescribing another active ingredient for the new symptoms that had arisen.

What does the medication actually do to my body? The eczema medication, of course, goes to areas not affected by the eczema and the intestinal medication goes to places where it is not needed – what is the effect of the medication in those areas? Is my body able to distinguish what goes where?

Each doctor is only responsible for one area of my body; just as if I were made up of individual parts. But he prescribes medication to me that usually affects my entire body. I find it shocking that five doctors, without consulting with each other, are working on my "individual parts".

Since the side effects usually only manifest themselves, can be felt or can be seen in one organ or body part, I have to go and see a different doctor each time. So the doctor I have seen previously rarely finds out whether what he has prescribed has actually worked. How can I manage this?

It would be easier if I could be treated as a whole person by just ONE doctor. A doctor who knows me, who is responsible for the stomach and intestines, the skin and hair and for both headaches and back pain – and who can also cure everything. He could happily consult with specialists when it comes to laboratory or x-ray findings. I think that on the search for the causes of the illness, more progress would be made this way and doctors would be more interested in finding a cure.

At the end of October, I had another appointment for an endoscopy; this would determine whether the clinical progression of the colitis had improved. "Interval with no bleeding. Ulceration of the rectum found to be in remission, subsequent continuation of Salofalk treatment, at least 3x500 mg for a further six months." were the findings.

The effect of the cortisone directly on the intestines is obviously more effective than in tablet form. The type of foam, with its large surface area, also caused no problems for me since it did not create any added pressure on the intestines.

But what had caused the skin problems on my face? Is the medication helping me, even though I don't tolerate it very well? Is it not suitable for me? The scalp eczema was getting worse even though the cortisone had been stopped; this was now being treated with Terzolin.

However, the Terzolin had obviously been responsible for the stomach pains that started in November. My GP now diagnosed gastritis.

Worries became everyday life. Helmut became virtually my only source of solace. But with so much going through my head, I didn't want to burden him. The only contact I had with my friends was mainly at birthdays and then we had other things to talk about. I didn't want to talk about my illness. What am I meant to say sitting there at the coffee table? Where am I meant to go with my thoughts, feelings, difficulties, problems and questions? Is it possible that so many people have been suffering with this condition for decades and that there are still no answers to all these questions?

I tried to avoid any form of stress and overexertion in my daily work, during severe flare-ups, in order not to provide the disease any points of attack. I not only reduced all human contact to a minimum, but also further reduced other activities. I assumed this would work like a process of elimination. Eventually, if I don't do anything anymore, don't move anymore, the illness will have no cause anymore, and then I will feel better. But by doing so, am I not wasting my life; the most precious thing I have? Wouldn't the opposite make more sense? Should I not enjoy living life to the full? Should I think less, do more and just let nature take its course? Why can't I shake everything off and just get going? What is stopping me living my life? Am I the obstacle?

A request for counselling

I wished that, in addition to treating the symptoms of the disease, there was also psycho-social counselling on hand, life coaching, together with family members too. What my life will look like in a few years from now when this disease has progressed further is a question I ask myself, especially when a new flare-up brings my mental state down again. That's when I start to fear for the future. When will I have to have my first surgery, how will I live with a stoma? How will I make a living if I am increasingly unable to work? Will the family cope? How will my children's lives be affected by this? And, above all, will I become a burden to my family? I feel as if my life were a tear-off calendar, the illness tearing a sheet off each day and throwing it away, unused. When will it stop?

My doctors appear to be overwhelmed by my questions. They have as little training in the psycho-social field as they do in nutritional issues. This creates frustration and helplessness, and the feeling of being overwhelmed continues to increase. You have to cope with everyday life yourself, but at best there are medicines for this too. My health insurance company pays for the medication and my doctor's appointments.

But who can give me advice about how I can manage my life again? Who can make me healthy again? I feel like I've been abandoned with these issues. At that time, I also knew nothing about the existence of self-help groups or patient organisations and received no information or practical help from my doctors.

Lots of little white lies had become part of my daily life now. Not only would I try to respond to the question of how I was, especially in my working life, with fair-weather answers so that I didn't lose loyal clients, but I would also answer questions of why I was too early or too late, why I suddenly had to leave or couldn't wait, with fanciful excuses and fibs. I didn't want anybody to know the truth.

My condition was often an enormous challenge for Helmut. I could never say when I would be ready to work in the office and what I would be able to do during the day. Nevertheless, he always remained calm, organised and worked. He postponed deadlines where possible, took over my jobs when they were urgent and took care of the apprentices' projects.
Our company's order situation was ideal. We didn't have to worry about orders, they came from recommendations. Our portfolio was impressive. Years ago, I could never have dreamed of the projects that we developed and designed each month. We now had four apprentices and four colleagues in the company and since we now offered website design as part of our range of services, we needed to recruit more experts.

But how was I meant to cope with these challenges now, in my state? I used the weekends to look through and correct the current orders in peace or to prepare new projects so thoroughly that the employees could start on them on the following Monday. It was quiet in the office at the weekends and I worked as long as my body would physically allow me to. There was no pressure if I need to use the toilet. There was nobody there to feel embarrassed with and there were no telephone calls. I now found it very difficult to work several consecutive hours, my body needed to move. When I sat for long periods of time, I felt the burning sensation increase as acids were building up in my gut. If the telephone rang, I felt it as stress. Luckily, it was usually only Helmut who was wanting to know how I was doing.

Making calls becomes impossible

I'd been having problems on the telephone for some time. A few years ago I assumed that this was caused by the radiation from the first mobile phones. Initially we had no landline connection and our first mobile phone had a very high transmission power, because the networks were not yet very well developed. Particularly when I was in the car and had to make many calls as a passenger, I would suddenly get stomach pains and would feel my heart racing. We haven't used this mobile phone for a few years now.

However, the following problem has now become an increasing burden: if I had to make a call, I would get stomach cramps followed by immediate diarrhoea. This wouldn't just happen on the mobile, but also when I had to make a call on the landline. Making calls had now become an added stress for me. I couldn't handle it: after picking up the receiver, I was able to speak a few sentences and then my entire body would break out in a sweat, the burning pain in my gut would then completely block my thoughts and render me incapable of responding in a coherent way. The urgency to empty my bowels would be so painful that I would have to bend double but I couldn't fight it. I would also be afraid that the noises that accompany this urgency and my groaning would be heard. I was often unable to interrupt the caller – who usually spoke immediately – quickly enough, despite the importance of grasping the key aspects of the matter in hand and offering an interim solution. However, I would still answer the phone because I always hoped that this next time I would be able to manage it. But time and again it overwhelmed me. As a result, I ultimately avoided answering the phone. My colleagues adapted to this.

Even today, though my intestines have healed, I am often the last person to answer the phone when it rings. I only ever use the mobile when I am travelling. I am still having to learn to use the phone again.

I am looking for something to help stabilise and calm me in these types of situations. I want to reach the stage where I no longer feel so shaken and then utterly exhausted and dead beat. It was when I was thinking about this that I remembered my biofeedback therapy. Maybe I could learn how to do it again and in turn help myself?

Biofeedback Therapy

It has been many years since I learnt about biofeedback on a course I attended. I tried to recall it. I hadn't forgotten the basic principles: relaxation, heaviness, warmth. I also tried to integrate my breathing and my heartbeat and as such relax. It worked really well, I was astonished how much came back to me. My body allowed itself to relax a little. I use this skill especially when I am in pain or when I can't sleep.
To make the most of it, I practised regularly. I would look for a quiet room, one that was as dark as possible, something comfortable to lie on and a warm blanket because I quickly get cold. If the environment was right, it was easier for me to relax. I was able to let go of myself, feeling relaxed, heavy and warm. My body would relax and the pain would lessen. It was often a resounding success: I could feel the pain reducing. This, in turn, was crucial for warming up, being able to fall asleep and ultimately finding tranquillity. Of course, it didn't work all the time. But the more I practised, the more successful I became at it. I never give up something quickly if I know what I'm doing is right. I had already bought myself a book with a CD about biofeedback to refresh my brain. If you're thinking of giving it a go, you should listen to the CD beforehand. I think it is important that the narrator has a pleasant voice.
If you can master the basic ritual after some time, it offers possibilities for further development through prescribed mantras. This allows you to influence specific problems subconsciously. I practised using the mantra: "My gut is pale pink, cool and relaxed", so I could visualise a situation of healing. Daily repetition over a long period of time can have a positive effect. But these mantras must follow specific rules. It is crucial that they are short and simple.
I have also had a positive experience with CDs for deep relaxation and with classical music for meditation. They are little periods of self-indulgence that I deliberately integrate several times a day as time-out. They allow me to switch off better and be at one with myself.

I think it is such a shame that not one of my doctors ever recommended biofeedback to me or prescribed a course. I figured this out for myself. The health insurance company probably wouldn't have financed it either. Once again, it was the holistic approach that I missed as a patient.

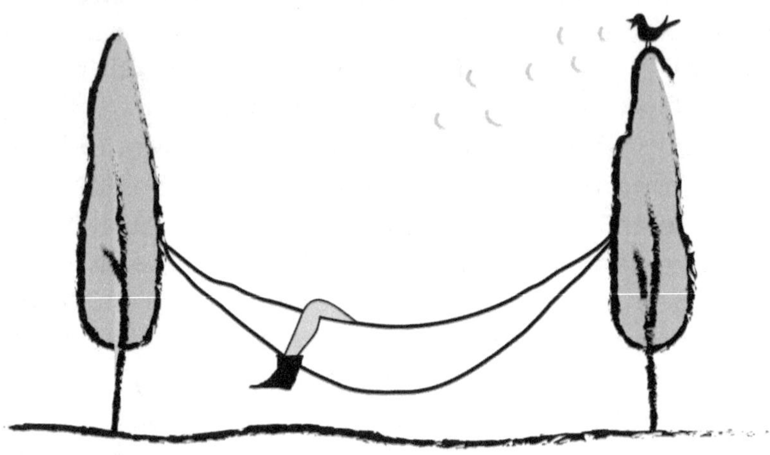

My hair loss and the scalp eczema had temporarily subsided. But these symptoms always came and went in phases. I wish I had some idea what the cause could've been for these. If something almost disappears, there must be a reason why it has got better. And when something breaks out again, there surely must be a reason for that too! I was still being prescribed Terzolin by the dermatologist.

In November, my gynaecologist referred me to a gastroenterologist for a colonoscopy. Will this tell me anything new? Will this doctor be able to help me? After all he's a specialist in this area. I was a little fearful of this examination because I imagined the colonoscopy to be very painful, given my current condition. The preparation for it was torturous in itself because this examination required the intestines to be "clean". To achieve this, I was given a laxative two days beforehand. In my already difficult situation, I felt this was an additional burden. Astonishingly, I remember very little about the examination itself. So I was all

the more surprised when the nurse told me after I woke that it was all over already.
Following the examination, the recommendation from the doctor was: "Continuation of the Salofalk treatment at 500mg at least 3 times a day, for a further six months due to ulcerative colitis currently being in remission.

Medication costs in 1998: 706,87 Euro

1999

Should I accept this illness?

The illness was sucking more and more out of my life. Will that change if I accept it? What does "accepting it" mean? Does it mean that I am in agreement with it and I should resign myself to it or does it mean that I have to recognise the current situation and fight for every little improvement?

Of course, I don't agree with it. A few short weeks of remission were not enough for me, especially since these phases were never completely pain-free. That is no trade-off because my life was like a nightmare. How can I say 'yes' to this daily nonsense? I would have to accept any progress of the disease. Because it had been getting worse with each flare-up. What was next? I wanted to change it, I wanted my old life back. I would do anything within my power to end this madness.

But I would probably have to learn how to accept the current situation as it stood. After all, it was just an illness. But I found it very hard, especially when a new flare-up started.
Often just a few sentences about work, projects, deadlines, a phone call or even a cool breeze would be enough to provoke colic-type pains that would cause my body to bend over double.
Some days I would put my coat on and then have to take it off again several times, I would sit in the car and then get out again, or I may have already driven halfway to work and then have to turn around again because my intestines seemed to be reeling! I had to work on creating a new measure of stability every day.
But the pain was becoming more and more unbearable. It was futile to hope that I would be able to control it consciously at some point.

The gas that would build up in my gut because of the inflammation just made the pain all the worse. The feeling that I was never actually "empty" had to be due to the swelling in the intestines. I ate barely anything and hardly dared to drink a sip. On days like these, I spent many hours on the toilet. I was cold, wrapped myself in a blanket and tried not to move in case I triggered more pain. Even at night, my bowel would not rest. When I finally got back into bed, I was so incredibly cold that I couldn't sleep and my body felt like an icicle. If I did fall asleep, after a short while, the pain would make me jump up. I would stumble from the bedroom, and everything would start all over again.

I read in a patient information leaflet for some medication that there was no cure for this condition. No doctor had actually said this to me before. But neither was there a discussion about the disease being curable during my consultation. Now that I was feeling so ill again, I was losing all hope of a normal life. My thoughts could only reach as far as the next intestinal spasm. I would be sitting on my sofa and all I could do was cry. I shook and was cold despite having a hot water bottle. I would just worry about any new cramp-like gripes tearing through me and forcing me to the toilet. I would squat there, cold, with stiffly frozen joints and muscles and I longed afterwards to simply return to my warm bed and fall asleep. The way back to bed seemed so far. I was completely zapped of energy, my body was going completely crazy. I had no strength left.

The happy moments are when the warmth returns to the bed and I am able to relax using my biofeedback training; the pain then noticeably eases.

The warmth gives me back some strength but then when I can't sleep, the frantic search begins again. What is it that keeps kicking my life so out of control? What's wrong in my life? What is different today than previously?

Or should the questions be: why is work of primary importance to me? It is important to always be up-to-date professionally? Can I give the rapidly increasing technical developments in communications the cold shoulder and still continue to work in this profession? Could I even just do nothing at all?

How will I learn to handle unpleasant situations better so that they don't lead to stress? How will I manage to stay relaxed now when there are deadline pressures and conflict situations? Tedious activities are tasks that have to be done but which must not burden my spirit because they are no more than the small building blocks of my daily work, tiny cogs in the bigger wheel. Am I able to learn this so that my body doesn't react to everything? Am I a particularly sensitive person? Is that my problem? Especially when I am weakened by the disease, I feel that the smallest of problems lead to major physical reactions. Even completely healthy people can react to conflict with diarrhoea or palpitations, that is well-known and is usually completely normal. I don't particularly recall having these problems in my life prior to being ill. Exam anxiety or stress didn't automatically mean that I needed to open my bowels. Now it is different, the simplest of daily demands lead to an immediate response. I react much more vehemently.

Talking about what is necessary: the call of nature

That is the fundamental problem of this condition. But why is it? For an infant, passing a bowel motion is a natural need, it knows no rules. Because "the call of nature" is a natural consequence of ingesting food. Metabolic end products must be ultimately excreted if we don't want anything to rupture.
The increasing ability of children to regulate their use of the toilet is rewarded by their families and society. Children are also taught that talking about bottoms and poops is not appropriate in many situations.

When we grow up, bowel movements become a taboo subject that we just don't talk about. False shame, imprinting and ignorance all arise from our upbringing. For adults, this part of the body functions normally, apart from if there is an infectious disease or poisoning of some kind. The loss of ability to control bowel movements with age is widely accepted as an inevitable evil.

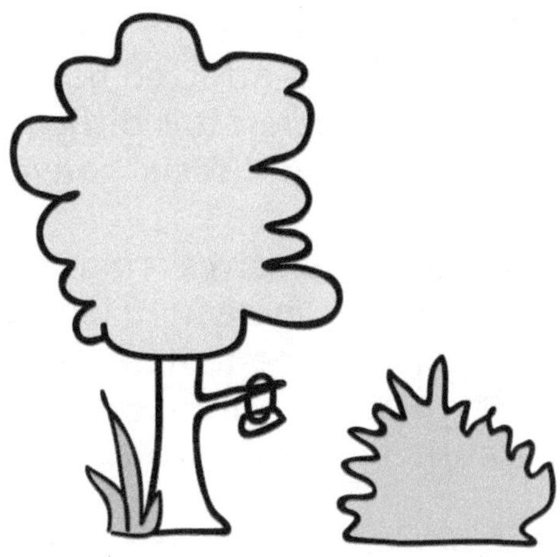

Dining is a culture. We like to eat stylishly and sophisticatedly. The subsequent call of nature is nowhere near as delightfully "celebrated". Our public toilet culture needs some development. The permanent dysfunction of an intestine that is still young and the problems associated with it are not known and only very few people are aware of it. Since they are always associated with unpleasant side effects, they are hardly ever addressed by those affected. The consequence is that frequent toilet visits with this condition are seen as a failure", especially if they are not the result of an upset stomach or an infection.
Flatulence is also a natural part of our digestive process. Though it is generally considered to be an imposition. The inflammation in the gut causes increased gas. Sometimes I felt like my stomach was just filled with air. How do I deal with the noises? Am I myself or is my body an imposition to others?
"If it doesn't make you fart or belch, you didn't enjoy it!" So they said at feasts in times gone by. That doesn't sound particularly desirable to me, but it does sound relaxed!
All this shows how much more difficult it is for those affected and for their families to talk to somebody about it. As a rule, it

is completely impossible to air and thus seek help with acute problems. So how can this be done better? I haven't found any definitive answers to this.

Although more has been published in recent years about ulcerative colitis and Crohn's disease, the main part of the discussion about the daily life of those affected has been restricted to private forums and family circles. It is difficult to break down the barriers that are built around social conventions and our own boundaries of modesty.

This is why we distance ourselves from other people and from life itself. In addition, with increasing illness in everyday life and in the professional environment, it becomes increasingly impossible to be among people. This leads to isolation. This didn't apply to me because my family protected me.

It is often not easy to deal with the disease and the resulting handicaps without losing self-respect. How do you do that? I had to learn here too to accept what I couldn't change. It wasn't me who determined my pace of life, it was my bowel. I didn't want to talk about it because I didn't want to burden others with my problems; it was burden enough for me; I feared for my acceptance. So I had to come up with some commonplace excuses and essentially lie to everyone around me. At best, I managed to organise my interactions in such a way that as few people as possible would notice. This is an additional burden that saps your strength and frays your nerves. So many acquaintances have said to me since I have been cured, "We had no idea that you were so poorly!" I have heard that so often, particularly now, many years later, in connection with this book. Helmut hadn't mentioned anything to others either and only rarely talked to anyone about it, because I hadn't wanted him to.

Nevertheless, it was important that I was able to speak out as often as possible about what I was feeling and experiencing. Despair needs an outlet. My family always offered a sympathetic ear. It is good if you have someone to listen to you. However, it is equally important to listen to your partner! Family members also need an outlet. This helps both sides learn to deal with embarrassing situations without causing discomfort. It is particularly helpful to see things from other perspectives. Discovering that the "embarrassments" that have become so stressful to you are accepted by your partner is a wonderful feeling. That's why I love you just the way you are! Wouldn't I do the same if it were the other way around? It is wonderful to have somebody that you can trust.

Not only are conversations important, but often you need unwavering help and support. I always had a guilty conscience if I was unable to say when I would be ready to go into the office. If we had joint meetings, Helmut would wait patiently for my "improvement" and for me to finally be able to get going. If it didn't work out, then he would drive me back again. He was always calm, took care of all the important things and allowed me to do my own thing. He was also there for the children, at breakfast time, to deal with their worries, clothes, jokes, school bags, quarrels, sports bags, washing, broken bikes and all preparations concerning the office or deadlines. Despite this, I felt the approaching deadline pressure. Time and again, when I had my coat on, and again when I finally got in the car, my bowel would make its presence felt. He would then often have to drive in to work alone and he would be late.
Where did he get the patience and strength from? He never blamed me or intentionally placed pressure on me. He always calmed me and only ever had kind words and would take me in his arms. So much peace. So much suffering. My feeling of having failed again was somewhat compensated by this.

In March, I had another appointment with my doctor. Of course, each time there was the full rigmarole: take bloods, partial and full blood counts, iron level check due to the high blood loss, urine analysis and proctoscopy.
The nurses were very friendly and I wasn't stressed. However, the examination was never particularly pleasant. The laboratory confirmed the diagnosis of: "Abundant discharge of pus, no indication of malignancy". So no improvement but no serious deterioration either.
In addition to the Salofalk tablets, I was given Salofalk enemas.

One enema (rectal enema) contains four grams of mesalazine. Application is easy thanks to the practical packaging. I was also given cortisone in the form of Colifoam rectal foam. The advantage of this was that the cortisone could reach the affected areas directly. This puts less strain on the body and does not affect your appetite as severely. Because of the anaemia, I was given Ferro Sanol capsules, an iron preparation.

After two weeks, I was feeling significantly better and I was able to reduce the cortisone. I was now using the Colifoam rectal foam and Salofalk enemas alternately so that the cortisone could slowly be flushed out of my system. After four weeks I continued to be treated with the Salofalk enemas with the aim of achieving a state of remission. I was prescribed vitamin E for the rheumatic pains in my hip joints as well as in my hands. I felt like it made me more stable and motivated to cope with everyday life. I felt more balanced as a result. The health insurance company paid for it all, which I was very grateful for.

My family gave me strength during these periods. I particularly loved and enjoyed the effervescent nature of my daughters. They coped with school very independently, helped in the house and they argued a lot! But shortly after, I would hear them cackling, giggling and playing together having fun and sharing secrets. It was wonderful to see how they got on with each other. I hope that later in life they will have a similar affectionate and honest relationship as I have today with my sister.

I cooked lunch for the children every day. For school, they took sandwiches and fruit, along with some small sweet treat each day in their lunchboxes. All parents did this, I thought. The children would be so happy when they opened their lunchboxes at break-time to find a little surprise in there. They would know that I was thinking of them and love them.

Much is different these days, especially as far as nutrition is concerned as I know all too well coming from the days of the former East Germany. There are a lot more temptations, often containing artificial additives. Could that have played a role? Have I perhaps not tolerated "reunification" in terms of food technology? If so, how could I find out what doesn't agree with me?

During a flare-up, I tried to eat puréed carrot or mashed potato, onions or oats in warm milk, pasta or chicken soup. Everything is cooked as carefully as possible, a lot is puréed. I felt no relief from this nor did I feel any better. Perhaps it would be even worse with a different diet? My mother recommended that I eat processed baby food out of jars. I had no success with that either. It was actually no different to my own puréed vegetables and I had already raised my children on this. Do I know if I'm feeding my children properly? What is a good diet? Who can tell me more about it?

My bicycle seems to understand me

Spring was finally here. It was a Sunday and the weather was wonderful. I had overcome my morning ailments, my bowel was calm, which relaxed me. I therefore wanted to do something that would benefit me so I planned to go on a bike ride. I rode in the direction of the fields and enjoyed the warmth of the sun and the smell of spring. I was doing really well so I extended the circuit further than I had planned. When I returned from my excursion, I noticed that the rest of the day was surprisingly pleasant and that I felt fine. I noticed a distinct difference I didn't have to go to the toilet after the bike ride and I felt a complete peace even after eating dinner! This pleasant feeling took me by surprise. I happily took that little slice of life that was offered to me: feeling a little overconfident, I thought I would cycle to work on Monday. Should I risk it? In any event, the weather was not going to stop me. So on Monday, I set off. Shorts, T-shirt, no breakfast. My commute took me predominantly through woods and meadows, across a moorland and an industrial park with cycle paths. The route was about eight kilometres and barely frequented. Since I scarcely came across anybody, it would not have been a disaster if my bowel had decided to make its presence felt. This thought gave me the confidence I needed. Everything went swimmingly! I was very proud of myself when I arrived at the office, I felt really well and got straight on with my work. By lunchtime, I had achieved so much and was amazed at how well I was still doing. I noticed that I had no problems throughout the entire morning. I neither had to go to the toilet, nor did I have any pain. My hypersensitive bowel was not active and I was even able eat.

However, I started with mild pain that afternoon. As I went to the toilet again for the first time, I thought: here we go again! If I don't get on my bike now, the pain will continue to increase! If I wait too long, I won't be able to get out of here on my bike! So I packed up my things and off I went. It worked! As soon as I sat on my bike and rode a short distance, my bowel calmed down, and a pleasant feeling spread throughout my body. When I arrived home, I was pretty wiped out because of the unusual strain of the day, but all-in-all I was fine!

What an interesting experience. So this was how it was going to be. From now on, I would cycle to the office every morning and cycle back again every afternoon.

Sitting on my bike immediately after getting up meant that, in a sense, I was able to "trick" my sensitive morning bowel almost every day. The movement, oxygen, improved breathing when pedalling, the relaxed thoughts when riding, enjoying nature, the peace ... whatever it was, my bowel relaxed.

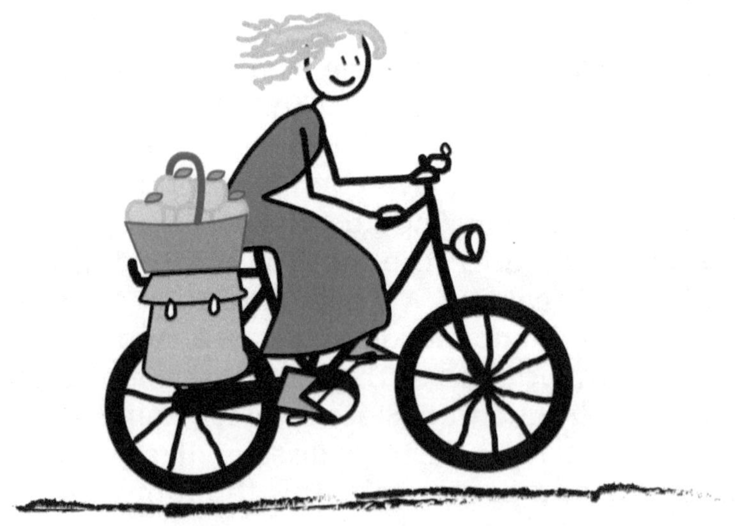

So I got used to working intensively in the morning and as soon as the first pains started, I packed up the work I had already done and rode home. It wasn't always easy, the work wasn't geared to my well-being, but for me it was a huge win!
I cycled in all weathers, even in the rain or when it was cold, because I realised that I couldn't stop! If I didn't ride my bike, the problems would return! I was dependent on my bike rides. The illness had not been cured by them but the symptoms had been noticeably reduced. But why had no doctor suggested this? Do they know anything about its effects?

Alternative practitioners
and living intestinal bacteria

I am always on the lookout for information that could help me. So I started to develop an interest in alternative healing methods. In my area, there was an alternative practitioner who I wanted to get some advice from. So I arranged an appointment to see her.
She spent a good hour with me and wanted to know a lot about my life. She made detailed notes from our conversation. This in itself was clearly different from my previous treatment with the specialist.
With the help of a metal pen, which had a small ball on the head, she measured the currents on the tip of my index finger. The persistent pressure was very unpleasant for me.
As a result of the measurement and the conversation, she recommended that I change my diet by completely avoiding certain things. These included: pineapples, pears, buttermilk, currants, quark, margarine, cod, sole, halibut, tuna, fermented milk and milk. So some fruits, several dairy products and saltwater fish. Margarine was also included, though I don't eat this anyway as I don't like it. She also prescribed me a large bag of herbal tea, which was made up for me at the chemist as per her instructions. She also started me on Bach flower remedies, which I was to use for a few months. After the next consulta-

tion, chocolate and all other sugary foods were added to the list of foods I had to avoid. My health insurance company would not bear the costs of the treatment and prescribed products as well. But I knew this beforehand.
I changed a lot of things as a result and cooked and lived according to these rules for several weeks. The foods mentioned were completely eliminated from my meal plan. I purchased the prescribed remedies from the chemist.

At about the same time I also talked to my gynaecologist, who always had time and understanding for my questions and problems, and I told her that I was also being treated by an alternative practitioner. I assumed she would be sceptical and was surprised when she actually encouraged me to try alternative approaches. She said that since the cause of the illness is unknown, there could be individual solutions that may bring some relief. I found that really uplifting because I felt that she was giving my illness the necessary attention and that she really wanted to help me find a way out. I felt acknowledged as a patient because I was able to play an active role in my own treatment.

She also had another idea, however, which was: E. coli Nissle – living intestinal bacteria – which was intended to help the flora in my gut to "reorganise" itself and thus to heal. That gave me new hope. I thought this was a great suggestion. It sounded logical to me: Sick intestinal bacteria that works against my own body and destroys the gut are replaced by healthy bacteria that are good for my gut. This could support the treatment by the alternative practitioner, I thought. The beauty of it was that this medication is free from side effects. I found the description on the package insert to be informative so I will mention it here:
From the Mutaflor® (5201198) package insert: "… A functioning physiological intestinal flora is an essential characteristic of a healthy organism. The Escherichia coli bacterium associated with normal intestinal flora, of which a particular strain (E. Coli NISSLE 1917) is contained in MUTA- FLOR®, plays a key role. Its ability to create a viable environment for the majority of intesti-

nal bacteria through oxygen consumption is essential. It has strong antagonistic abilities against pathogenic micro-organisms and thus supports the barrier function of the physiological intestinal flora against invading foreign bacteria. Its metabolic products are vital sources of energy for the cells of the intestinal mucosa. The production of vitamin K covers, if necessary, the entire needs of humans. ..."

However, I couldn't detect any short-term, immediate reaction to this new treatment method. But two weeks later, we went on holiday. I was filled with hope that I would soon feel a positive effect thanks to these many new possibilities.

Holiday in Italy

With the Mutaflor®, my living intestinal bacteria, in the well-chilled glove compartment, Bach flowers, my tea mix and the Salofalk, I was ready to feel in full health in Tuscany. I wanted to enjoy this time to the fullest, spend a lot of time relaxing, so that the illness could finally have a rest itself. I saw this holiday as a huge opportunity. A romantic holiday home on a very large, secluded property with a pool was awaiting us. The location was wonderful. There were two families with plenty of room for everyone.

We cooked our own food. We bought local produce and delicacies. This meant that we could decide for ourselves what would appear on our plates. Our already grown-up children were, as always, included in the cooking and holiday plans, so I delegated the work which meant there was a lot of new inspiration.

I had brought my watercolours with me and looked for a good place to paint. The landscape provided a wonderful, romantic subject. The colours here were far brighter than at home, so painting was going to be a special experience. Once again, I found this hobby to be such a relaxing pastime, where I could completely switch off.

I roamed the forest around Florence with my sister-in-law. We fled from wild boars and overheard a musician preparing for a concert in a secluded woodland house. We made ourselves comfortable on a wayside and enjoyed the music. We applauded enthusiastically during the pauses and he leant out of his window and bowed. Then he disappeared on his Vespa with his violin and left the music-playing to the cicadas.

We went on excursions to the romantic cities of Florence, Siena, Perugia and Montepulciano. A particular highlight was the sulphur thermal baths in Saturnia. The actual source of the sulphur consisted of a small warm, winding stream and a waterfall. The current at the top of the waterfall was so strong that you had to hold on tightly to something if you were only very light in weight. A tuft of grass was enough to grab on to, your body fluttered in the warm water like a flag in the wind. I really enjoyed the relaxing feeling it gave me. Our car smelt devilishly good as we drove back home because we all had the smell of sulphur in our hair. I was pleased and happy and convinced that I was now on the up.

Up until the 7th day of the holiday, that was! Right in the middle of the holiday, my condition worsened. The pain increased and I couldn't get out of the bathroom in a morning. My bowel appeared distended and the bleeding was getting worse. As such, the only toilet for both families was occupied. I tried to get some rest during breakfast time but simply staggered back and forth between the toilet and bed.

What was wrong all of a sudden? I had carefully followed all the advice from my doctor and the practitioner. Why suddenly now, on holiday, when I have no stress? I was so upset about it. I had hoped that the much esteemed Mediterranean cooking would have supported the healing process.

Maybe a 14-day period was too short, perhaps my body hadn't had enough time to adapt to the changes? Or did relaxation and the holiday have nothing to do with it?

Perhaps the things that I had eaten to replace the foods I had to avoid weren't good for me? My practitioner had only told me what I should avoid, she hadn't told me what I was allowed to eat instead! On holiday in Italy, there was an overwhelming amount of pasta and pizza, Italian white bread, tomatoes, peppers, apricots, peaches, olives, salami, ham, cheese and wine. Which of these foods was not good for me?

Obviously, the intestinal bacteria were not able to keep the disease stable. It simply wasn't able to renew my intestinal flora and apparently didn't survive in my gut. Why not? Hope waned for me again. Each day of the holiday became more difficult, the activity of my illness stepped up a gear. So many new approaches, and no success!

Helpless

In September, after our holidays, I stopped riding my bike; my bowel simply wouldn't allow me to ride in the mornings anymore. The symptoms were much too great and increased by the day. A new, more violent flare-up began. This was now affecting the entire left, descending colon. I had never felt so weak and helpless. The feeling that my own body was destroying itself drove me to despair. The Salofalk was increased again to 3 x 1.5mg, which meant I was taking nine tablets per day. I was also started on steroid treatment in the form of Decortin tablets. The active ingredient in this is prednisolone. In the first week, I took 60mg, and from the second week onwards 40mg per day. Along with this I was prescribed Betnesol in enema form at night. One pouch of the ready-to-use solution contains 5mg of betamethasone.

By this point, I was feeling really sick. It was so bad that I was just sitting on the toilet, often I fell asleep completely exhausted from the pain, freezing and trembling, wrapped in a blanket, my legs drawn up and my arms wrapped around them. When I woke up, I tried to get back into bed, but it was even colder and my joints hurt terribly! I stopped eating, drank tea in small sips and was getting thinner by the day. I felt at the mercy of this disease.

I was also getting severe night sweats. Several times during the night, I would be drenched from head to toe. As a result, I would be freezing cold and I would endlessly put off changing my clothes and my bed covers. It was always the fear of the cold that stopped me. Sudden cold provoked an immediate cramp-like reaction in my intestines, which meant that I had to get out of bed again and I didn't know when I would be able to get back in and get warm again.

Signed off sick for the first time

I was signed off work sick from the middle of September. This was a new experience that I was having to adapt to for the first time.

As a self-employed person, you get your "salary" when you complete an order, write an invoice and the customer pays. If you don't work, you don't earn any money. But there are still overheads to be paid, for example, the office, insurance, national insurance contributions, taxes and of course living costs for the family.

It is therefore possible for a self-employed person to take out daily sickness benefit insurance. I had done that when I first became self-employed. To keep the costs as low as possible, I chose a tariff that after 14 days of sickness would compensate loss of earnings at a half daily rate and after four weeks at a full daily rate. The calculation is based on a minimum cost coverage. I thought the prospect of being sick for longer than four weeks would be very low. Basically, I only receive the full money for my livelihood after thirty days of sickness. Each sick note therefore presupposes that I can live on reserves for as long as possible. That was why I hadn't asked to be signed off sick before this.

This is complicated by the definition of a sick note by the health insurance companies. From the date of the sick note, I must no longer have any business-related contact with my office as this is regarded as a managerial activity and will lead to insurance benefits being withdrawn. In the event of sick leave, I had to sign the following commitment: "An unemployed person is considered to be a person who is unable in any way whatsoever to temporarily undertake his/her professional activities according to medical findings. Self-employed or freelancers must also not cooperate, manage or supervise". It is not taken into account that, as the company owner, I can't give up economic responsibility for my company. That was added stress for my business partner; he had to now undertake additional graphic design for customer orders and train the apprentices.

I now had to deal with a new task; that of my managing my illness. In order to stay on top of things, I set up a workspace at home for when I was off sick. It is very important to know and comply with all regulations and deadlines. The daily sickness allowance must be reapplied for with every visit to the doctor, but after 14 days at the latest. I only receive money if I complete this correctly. I had to also try to make fewer mistakes on days when I wasn't feeling so well.

There is a special form to complete for a sick note, which is to be extended regularly by the doctor treating me and sent promptly by me to the health insurance company. The doctor can invoice the cost for completing the form as an additional fee (DM 10.49), the patient must bear this cost because this is not part of the health insurance tariff and of course not part of the daily rate.

At the same time, all incoming invoices, for doctor's visits, lab tests and prescriptions, as well as the copying, filing and sending of originals to the health insurance company, must be checked and forwarded. In connection with this, payment receipts must be checked and the invoices always paid to the doctors on time.

I wasn't able to do this at first. It caused me stress and was hard for me because I had to explain the problem over the phone. My hope of being able to give up all my obligations for a few weeks due to the illness was dashed. I knew all the more now why I delayed being signed off sick for so long. But that is obviously the idea. I felt that was a huge burden in my situation. When you choose a health insurance company, you are usually quite young and healthy and you know nothing of the many details and challenges. After these experiences, I feel very disappointed about the role of the health insurance fund in my recovery. Of course a private health insurance company is a company and not a social welfare organisation. But wouldn't it be more efficient to do EVERYTHING possible to cure diseases for good for this very reason?

Good news

I was prescribed cortisone again. I was really concerned that this active ingredient would now be a constant companion of mine. This made me anxious. How will my body respond to it? But the strong cortisone treatment took effect again. The Decortin medication, an immuno-suppressant and a cortisone-based anti-inflammatory, had a significant impact. The inflammation regressed by the day. A new side effect for me thought was hyperactivity, which I had never experienced before. While taking the cortisone, I felt "wired" all day long. When I finally got to sleep at midnight, I would be up by four in the morning. Four hours sleep was enough for me and then I was wide awake. After a few weeks, once my bowel had calmed down, a 20-hour day was a walk in the park; I was hyperactive. So I would go for a walk at four in the morning through the meadows and across the fields. I watched the sunrise and experienced the waking of the day, enjoyed the daylight, the twittering of the birds and the fog over the fields. It was astonishing that my bowel did not send out any signals at this time. I had regained a piece of freedom, the medication had worked.
When we were discussing it in connection with this book, Helmut told me that he had had a different experience of the situation back then.
He found my constant mood swings and my hyperactivity as a huge additional burden.
But there were other side effects, including my unusually large appetite. I would get the urge to binge eat. I could polish off two full portions of dinner, one after the other, and for dessert,

I would stuff myself with two bananas. Even that would not make me feel full. Helmut found it astonishing what I could pack into my stomach. The natural consequences of this were that, after a few weeks, I couldn't fit into my trousers anymore, not to mention my suits and dresses. I developed a moon face and gained ten kilos. But I was on the up! The findings at the end of September confirmed this. (Still areas of inflammation in the sigmoid, UC seen to be healing). The Decortin was therefore reduced at intervals of 14 days to 30mg initially and then to 20mg. Alongside this, I also used Betnesol rectal instillation and Salofalk enemas on alternate days. I was also prescribed ferritin to help my iron levels to recover.

My recovery was not only monitored by my doctors, but also by the health insurance company. The company carried out home visits. Though in truth I suspected that this wasn't really about the condition of my health but rather about checking that I had complied with the aforementioned agreement. I became aware of this when Helmut told me that my office had repeatedly been the first point of contact for the representative of the health insurance company. He had asked the staff about my attendance at the office.

At the start of October, I was only taking 20mg of Decortin. I felt a little more stable. My sick leave ended, but as well as a feeling of insecurity, I now had a relaxed feeling of relief and relief from pressure and many obligations.

As I went back to work again, a new surprise awaited me: I couldn't see properly. I suffered with dry, itchy eyes. Could this possibly be linked to the long-term cortisone treatment? Working on the screen was a disaster for me because everything would simply blur in front of my eyes. I also felt that as soon as I opened my eyes, they were full of fine fluff, this led to my touching and rubbing them. Every touch made my already reddened eyes worse. The eye doctor prescribed me Artelac eye drops, which were supposed to act as a tear substitute. What had happened to my tears?

At the end of October, my course of Decortin was extended by four weeks as the bleeding had suddenly appeared again. Because, during these weeks, I had increasingly suffered with severe cramping in my legs, I was also prescribed magnesium.

An unexpected problem was also my dry mouth, it was as if my tongue was stuck and could not move. It was a most unpleasant feeling. I tried to help myself by drinking constantly. Saliva is of course vital for digestion, would this cause me more problems? That gave me cause for concern. Why were all my mucous membranes so dry?

I was able to reduce the Salofalk to 3x2 tablets by the end of the year. This is actually the highest dose, as far as I could deduce from the package insert. ("... For acute treatment ... as directed by the doctor, the daily dose can be increased to two tablets three times a day depending on the response to the medication and on individual needs.")

I felt considerably better. If I was able to relax in the mornings, after a few visits to the toilet, I would then usually be able to make it to the office without any problems. However, I felt exhausted during this time and the daily worry of not being able to complete my work within the specified time frame was a constant weight on my shoulders. I was now finding it very difficult to take on the responsibility for any ongoing projects.

I also had to seek out new business because word-of-mouth advertising only worked if you were always around. However, I just didn't have the strength for it.

I became increasingly anxious about no longer being able to cope to the daily demands. I no longer saw new projects as a way of securing the order situation for the coming weeks, which used to trigger feelings of happiness and satisfaction in me. Instead I became anxious that I wouldn't cope with these additional projects because I didn't have enough strength. And that would cause even more pressure.

It would be so great if I could just have a prolonged period of calm and the disease would regress. I just wanted to live. So I could finally have time for my family again and could take care of the development of my office. I would really love just a snapshot of real life again!

Amalgam

Out of worry that this period of rest may only be temporary, I started to think more deeply about how to prevent a new flare-up. At the same time, I also received information about the role of amalgam in chronic inflammatory bowel diseases.
Can fillings play a role in an illness? Are they poisoning my body? Perhaps the fillings that I had in my youth are no longer alright? I resolved to research this in more detail and spoke to a dentist about it. She convinced me to gradually have my fillings removed; my dental fillings were already a few years old anyway, she said. She proposed proceeding carefully and using a rubber dam to prevent toxins from infiltrating the body. In addition, medication containing ingredients such as zinc and selenium should support detoxification.
I decided to go for this treatment while I was feeling better. Maybe the outcome would be so successful that it would prevent a new outbreak of the illness? This option seemed like a hopeful one to me and I clung onto it. If the fillings are the cause, maybe I would be cured?
The treatment dragged on over several months. My amalgam fillings were removed. At this time, I felt reasonably well, the symptoms were bearable. Though I do recall that the toilet in the dental practice was increasingly a port of call for me, even several times during the treatment itself. During this time, my bowel was unstable, but I had no bleeding. I saw this as a sufficient and promising prerequisite.

I want to do something for myself!

A remission phase is also a time for me to reflect on how to proceed and how I would like to be able to cope with lots of different things in the future. I couldn't be sure in any way that this relative calm period would be long-lasting.
At the start of my illness, I was convinced a doctor would prescribe me medication and that would make me healthy again.

Now I know that the medication will not make me well but will only provide some help by suppressing an acute flare-up. I also know that I am only one of many patients for my doctor and each individual patient is only given a small amount of time. It was therefore important to use this time effectively. I wanted to learn more from my doctor to further my knowledge. In the meantime, I had learnt to ask questions until I understood everything properly. It was my right, particularly since I was paying for this information. I always have the feeling that people want to "spare" me the necessary explanations or that the effort to explain things was too much or that one doctor or another didn't have the relevant information and would have to look for it somewhere first.

Initially, I thought that doctors cured many people in their professional lives and therefore had a wealth of personal experience in treating patients with this condition. But when I left the consultation room, I often felt that something had been forgotten or disregarded. I felt like I was being processed according to a pattern. I was bemused by the fact that, at the end of the treatments, either a new medication would be prescribed or the dose of an existing one adjusted. I missed the alternatives and I particularly missed the opportunity of being able to do something for myself; I wanted to be included in my own recovery. For example, if I had to tread water every day in order to strengthen my immune system, I would do it. If I had to wear gloves in the future when doing the housework to avoid any damage, then I would do that too but there were never any concrete instructions for me.

I handed the prescription in, travelled home and I didn't know what to do to help myself, how I could support, strengthen and pamper my body. A heat cushion? A herbal compress? A specific herb or spice, healing mud, exercises? Everything depended solely on the medication and I couldn't do anything myself! I felt like I wasn't part of it. My task was restricted to "obeying" and my studies were confined to the package insert leaflet.

What is it again that the small print says so eloquently? For the risks and side effects, read the package insert and ask your doctor or pharmacist. I had lots of questions to ask, but no doctor could answer them for me. For example: can I prevent any of the side effects from the medication? Which household remedies could relieve them, which alternative applications could stabilise my condition? I don't want to be continually caught off guard by 'apparitions' which I had never even dreamed of until now. Or: why doesn't my body fight back anymore, like it used to be able to? When and why did it stop? What are my body's weak spots and how can I strengthen them? What is my immune system lacking? Have disruptions to the system accumulated over a long period of time, until the barrel has overflowed, so to speak? What can I do to change the course of the illness and finally get better? So many questions, but where do I find the answers?

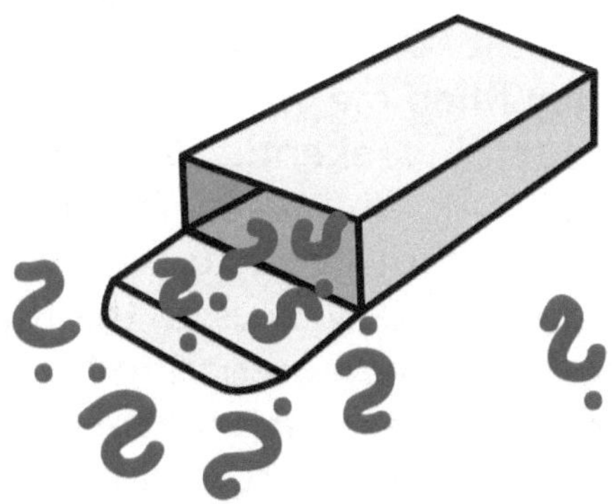

What I was missing was a doctor who would ask me what it was that I needed as a person? What was going wrong in my life? It was the holistic approach that I was missing, I know that now. How much time do you devote to yourself on a daily basis? When will I learn that it isn't a crime to give yourself some self-care? It doesn't make me a bad person if I can't cope with something or if I need help. The opposite is true, it is bad thing not to think of yourself. However, I was still not willing to lower the demands I placed on myself and to adjust them to my current situation. Consequently, I was always running around on empty. That was bound to have consequences!

Medication costs in 1999: 1355.99 Euro

2000

Filled with hope

In February I turn 40. Has half of my life passed already? If it has, how does it feel? In my head, I still feel like a little girl. That's a reason to celebrate, but how? How will I celebrate my birthday?

Physically, I felt frail. I was running to the toilet 15 to 25 times a day. This made me feel depressed and disheartened. I believed that pain was now likely to be a permanent fixture in my life.

I neither wanted a stressful birthday nor a small party with the obligations that came with it. The thought of organising and "getting through" the day filled me with anxiety.

I just wanted a long, peaceful weekend. We decided to spend a couple of days in the Thuringian Forest. The journey wasn't too long and it would do Helmut good to get away, too. Our youngest daughter, Josefine, came with us on the trip. Franziska was already 18 at this point and was preparing for her A-levels, so she wanted to stay at home. A somewhat secluded holiday home was ideal, and I could face my "constant commitments" with a sense of calm. My family, rest and exercise in the fresh air was just what we needed. The holiday home had a little kitchen so that we could cater for ourselves. We spent a long of time playing the game "Settlers of Catan" because our "Finchen" loved this game and enjoyed the fact that we were using the time to "settle" together. On the Sunday of my birthday, we went for a walk. I received a lot of phone calls which made me very happy. But nobody knew or could have guessed how difficult every conversation was for me and what consequences it often had. The forest offered me the protection and security that I needed and in the end I was more than happy to receive every single one of the calls!

What will this year bring for us? We had lots of plans, we wanted to build our own family home. We purchased the plot of land last year. We were going to build a house with a large kitchen and with a bedroom for each child. At the start of April, the building work began and we were of course completely elated and filled with ideas.

By the end of February, my condition had had enough rest and made its presence felt with renewed vigour. The pain got worse and I lost an increasing amount of blood. My body responded with the usual tiredness and exhaustion. These painful highs and lows of the illness made planning life impossible. How bad would it be this time? I had to go to the doctor, I needed a different medication. I had given up all hope of my body's slow detoxification following removal of the amalgam and, with it, any slow eradication of the disease. What I had hoped for several months crumbled away in just a few days. This pained me as the despair came through the same door as the illness. The amalgam was just one cog in the big wheel of many causes of the condition. I could only work on a sporadic basis now, usually at the weekends. Where possible, I avoided contact with my staff and often only went in in the evenings when my colleagues had left the office. I felt better working through into the night, doing whatever I could do. Those urgent jobs needed to be done, provided my strength held out. I slept wherever I slumped, sometimes even on the office floor.

This flare-up was treated with Betnesol enemas. Using these was more unpleasant than taking the tablets. The side effects were completely different. Whereas previous medication had led to my feeling more energetic, I was now tired and lethargic. I slept practically the entire day. Increasingly I noticed less of what was happening around me. I was only awake when I had to go to the toilet. I would warm myself up again with hot tea and my hot water bottle. My biofeedback training helped me to fall asleep again. But the medication worked. After 14 days, I started to show a marked improvement.

A new side effect was the now severe muscle cramps and they were indeed significantly worse than I had ever known them to be. They affected both legs, feet and my buttocks. It was very difficult to get on my feet feeling like this because I could only use my arms to bring myself to a secure footing. The attacks came several times a day and also several times during the night, in the middle of my sleep when I would wake up, flailing around and helplessly crying out. The pain was excruciating and it was difficult to stay upright. Most of the time, I had absolutely no control over my body, especially if it was also affecting my buttocks, it became a rather sporadic affair. An unpleasant consequence of this of course was the muscle soreness the following day. I found this all so disheartening. I took magnesium to relieve the cramps. The health insurance bore the cost of this. Then the joint problems started again. My elbows and knees no longer wanted to play ball. I stood in front of the stairs and I was unable to get up the steps alone, not even with the aid of the banister. I needed help to do this. At the office, Helmut had to carry me over the back door step. By the middle of April, the cortisone treatment came to a successful end and the symptoms improved. But of course the next problem was just around the corner. My skin problems were back again. The previously mentioned oozing eczema on my head broke out. My scalp was sticky, weeping and crusty. I also had dry eczema on the right side of my face. When making facial expressions, more and more individual areas would split open, the oozing fluid would then crust over and lead to further tension. The port wine stain on my neck returned in all its glory (it had never truly disappeared this entire time). I was now also plagued by very unpleasant anal eczema that I tried to relieve by taking Sitz baths. I was in despair. I sat around the house, didn't dare to venture outside in public and couldn't even cry because any facial movement would cause my skin to split.

I was prescribed lots of ointments and drugs by the dermatologist: Ichtoderm cream and Ichthoseptal solution, Proctoparf ointment, zinc oxide ointment, Remederm cream, Widmer and Tamnolact gel.

I looked at this collection, baffled. I asked myself why there were so many different ointments for the head, face, neck; basically an ointment for each area of the skin? The cause of my skin irritation is obviously the same. They always started at the same time, usually during or after being treated with cortisone. And isn't skin just skin? Is the structure and functioning of the skin not, to a great extent, the same? What does my skin need now?

I reflected again on why there was a different doctor for every part of the body. Is it possible to treat a person when you are only interested in the bowel? Or the scalp? That can't be possible, the body is a perfectly coordinated network.
It is important for me to make decisions about my medication and also my treatment. I am not made in such a way that I can allow somebody else to make a decision about me and my body and I can't simply do as I am told without asking questions. It doesn't work like that. I want to hear alternatives from my doctor. My body belongs to me, I am therefore responsible for it and consequently should have a say.
I'm getting more suspicious of the system with each new experience. I keep getting the feeling that no one is really interested in my healing. As a chronically ill person, am I perhaps simply a good customer?

Where can I get information from?

I didn't know of any books on the subject at the time. The Internet was just starting to emerge. The only thing I had were the brochures produced by the pharmaceutical companies for patients and doctors. These days it is much easier, but are we getting the correct information?

In a patient information leaflet from Alfred-Nissle, entitled "*Intestinal flora and chronic inflammatory bowel disorders*" from 1998, I read the following on the subject "*Intestinal flora and the immune system*": "*... Normal, healthy intestinal flora plays a very significant role in the development of the immune system because this harmless bacteria activates and trains the immune cells to prepare them to defend against invading pathogens.*

Without healthy intestinal flora, the functioning of the immune system cannot be maintained. "
It made me think: maybe my immune system is sick because my intestinal flora is not healthy, or is this not healthy because my immune system is not functioning correctly? Which problem came first? And why did the Coli bacteria not help? What is wrong with my intestinal flora?
I continued reading: "… Not least, intestinal flora plays a role in digestion especially in the breaking down of fibre which is so important for the colon (e.g. cell walls of fruit, vegetables and bran), which cannot be broken down by the body's own digestive enzymes. They are therefore transported to the colon unchanged. Previously it was incorrectly thought that these were not necessary fibre for the body.
The metabolites which produce the intestinal bacteria from this fibre are however crucial for feeding the cells of the intestinal mucosa. There are so-called short-chain carboxylic acids, acetic acid, propionic acid, butyric acid and lactic acid. These bacterial metabolites are very rich in energy. In connection with chronic inflammatory bowel disorders, they play a special role because if they are unable to store energy, feeding the mucosa cells is not properly guaranteed and it can lead to the cells dying off prematurely and therefore the mucosa becomes inflamed.

I found this interesting. Why hadn't my doctor explained this? Up until now, no doctor had recommended that I increase my intake of fruit, vegetables and bran to make my mucous membranes healthy. It was clearly recommended in this brochure! Was I supposed to be eating dietary fibres after all? Until now, a low-fibre diet had been the right thing to protect my intestines. Rice, oatmeal, mashed potato, rusk, pasta, semolina, pastries, cooked vegetables, puréed vegetables, vegetable soups, lean dairy products, sausages and lean meat, all cooked gently – but to my understanding this is the exact opposite! How is this contradiction possible? It said here that I didn't actually need any medication, I needed fruit, vegetables and bran! Had this information been deliberately withheld from me? Should I now be eating fibre-rich foods to protect my gut, or will these things damage my poorly intestines? Does the previously recommended diet contain sufficient dietary fibres? I don't think so. Who can I ask? Who will give me the right answer?

The eczema had marred my face for several months. When things got better for a few days, I would get my hopes up, but then it would break out again and the whole cycle would start over; this included the appearance of the port-wine stain on my neck. At the point at which it went a deep red colour, the skin would split open. The fluid would then run down my neck and crust over. If I tried to dab it with water, my skin would react with extreme dryness and stress. I got skilled at wrapping my neck in sterile, cotton kitchen towels as scarves. The port-wine stain changed in intensity daily, it would go from a delicate pink then suddenly back to a deep red again. In the meantime, I was despairing in the belief that this would stay with me throughout my entire life, like a huge unsightly liver spot. I found that idea frightful. I felt completely disfigured by it.

This port-wine stain was treated with Dermatop ointment, Rp. Leuchkichthyol, Aquapurif., Proctofoam HC Susp. N1, Basiscreme DAC (base cream), cod liver oil ointment and various other manufactured ointments. It took several months before my skin looked normal again. For a long time, I got used to looking at myself in the mirror on a daily basis, checking to see whether it was appearing again. I was always expecting it to come back. It felt so good to have my face back! What a wonderful feeling it was to have smooth, close-textured skin. However, the port-wine stain on my neck often reared its head time and again. As big as a red light, forever shining.

In April, my gastroenterologist recommended that I apply to the health insurance company for frankincense therapy (H 15 Ayurmedica). He had learned about it himself and gave me the material to study, hoping that this active ingredient would help me further. "It is a brand new therapy, not yet well-known in Germany. There are many promising studies on it", he said and gave me an informal letter that also detailed a cost estimate. I got the impression that this specialist was up-to-date with the latest research findings and was well-informed. So, I applied to the health insurance company for reimbursement of the costs. Because I hadn't expected a speedy response to my application, I started the treatment filled with hope. It was something new, perhaps this medication would help me further. So, I didn't want to lose any time. The pharmacy bought the drug in from Switzerland.

Six weeks later, I received the refusal to reimburse costs from the health insurance company. "… since there was insufficient evidence of effectiveness due to a lack of studies …" The treatment was planned for a year. The costs would run to around 4000 Euros. At this time, the medication was not yet authorised for use in Germany. After three months, I had to stop the treatment for cost reasons. There was no way I could guarantee a positive impact in the short term. My condition had not changed during this period but fortunately, there were no side effects. I still had particular problems in the mornings, coupled with pain. Over the duration of the day, it regulated itself to fewer, albeit painful, toilet visits. I longed for a period where my body could feel at ease, where I could simply go about my daily work undisturbed. I wanted to laugh again in a carefree manner.

Another new medication that I was prescribed was Duspatal lozenges. They were intended to have an anti-spasmodic effect on the bowel and as such reduce the level of pain. They relaxed the bowel and had a rapid effect. They were very helpful, especially when it came to sleeping. I also had no side effects from them.

The colitis cycle

I don't know exactly when it started but, for weeks, my colitis had a 2-day cycle. This cycle was so regular that I was able to adjust my deadlines around it. One day I'd be well and the following day I'd be ill; it went on like this for some time. How was this possible?

All the pain, bleeding and persistent toilet visits completely disappeared. I could eat normally and only rarely went to the toilet which was pain-free. On these days it was possible to stick to my deadlines, to focus on my work orders and to look after the house. Driving the car was also not a problem for me. But then the next day was hell. It started early in the morning. I felt like my gut was filled with acid – as if I had drunk a cup of household cleaner. That's how I imagined it; it burned, swelled and bubbled. It tore at me internally. I whimpered and bent over. Heavily wrapped up with my hot water bottles on my stomach and back, I crept under my blanket and didn't come out until the next time I had to run to the toilet. Always hoping that it would bring me some relief with the thought that perhaps some of this burning acid was leaving my body. I would return to bed weakened, shaking and freezing, like a wrung-out sponge. Again I built up all my lovingly-filled hot water bottles around me and tried to relax and accept their warmth. I tried to relieve the pain using biofeedback. On these days, I was grumpy and unfriendly with everyone. But I still got lots of help. A hot tea to warm me up was a small joy as well as being the only thing that I consumed on these days.

In the late afternoon, the pain would become more bearable, the burning reduced, the intervals between the cramps would get increasingly longer, until at some point calmness returned and I was able to fall asleep. In the evening, I would go for a walk, walk around the house, keep myself moving. I then felt considerably better. I had overcome it. I would be extremely hungry. My appetite would return and I'd looking forward to the opportunity of eating together with the family. The next day I would be better still, I was completely pain-free.
The day after that, it started all over again – the entire routine, the entire agony -, it went on like that for three months. I had no explanation for it but I was able to adjust to it. I could plan my time. The objective was to survive one day and then to start afresh on the second day. You really had to take this illness as it was and make the best of it.

Kohlrabi from my mother-in-law's garden

The summer holidays began and we travelled to Saxony for a weekend to visit my mother-in-law. On the Friday that we were leaving, I felt terrible again. I was a shivering bundle and didn't know what was going on around me. The only thing I knew was that I would feel better again by the evening and then we would be able to travel. I promised everyone, and so that's what we did. I looked forward to the Saturday because I knew I would feel better and we could all enjoy the day together. But what would happen on the Sunday when we had to travel back again? How would I get out of the bath in the morning and get into the car? How was I supposed to explain to Helmut's family what was wrong with me? Should I just say that I have diarrhoea? And how would I be in the car without a toilet and my warm cushions? It made me anxious. But I had to do it. Worrying wasn't going to help. The principle here is hope. It wasn't a round-the-world trip and Sunday was still a way off!

The family lived in a small village in Saxony. Just like a true farm, grandma had a small garden for vegetables and flowers. Of course, my mother-in-law knew that I often felt poorly and since she meant well, she gave me a huge, fresh kohlrabi on the Saturday! I peeled it immediately and took my time eating half of it. It was tender and juicy. Since I didn't know how my body would react to so much raw food, I decided to keep the other half for Sunday. Don't overdo it! A raw kohlrabi is undoubtedly healthy but would my bowel and the bleeding inflammation agree? I wanted to wait and see. I enjoyed the good Saxon cuisine with particular caution because there was always a lot of meat, a lot of sauces, dumplings and different kinds of cooked vegetables. For dessert, there was ice cream and various sweet drinks and iced teas. In the afternoons, we were served plenty of home-made cakes as well as shop-bought tarts. I was careful because the food I ate at home was different. I preferred tea to food, avoided roasted meat and sweet desserts because they didn't make me feel good. I tried to eat it what my bowel was accustomed to.

On the Sunday I woke expecting my usual bowel problems. But I immediately had a relaxed feeling: I felt well. I managed to get up, I ate a small amount at the breakfast table, always with the expectation that something would happen. But I still felt well even after eating breakfast. The first time in months, from one day to the next, the cycle had changed. I was pain-free for the second consecutive day and I hadn't needed to go to the toilet so often. This made me feel so relaxed. We could travel back without any problems. I was very happy that I had escaped the stress. I, of course, took my other half of kohlrabi with me and ate it on the journey back; I assumed by now that it wouldn't have a detrimental effect on me.

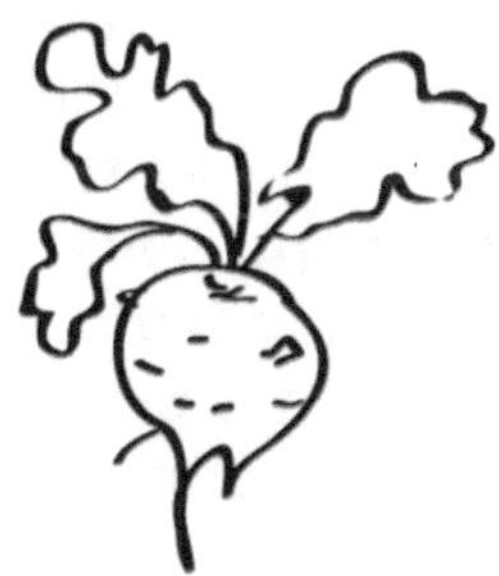

But now I had a new worry: how would I cope with work on Monday? My deadline planning was all over the place. Because on Monday, I was bound to be ill. I now had to operate on that assumption. It was important to me that I was able to do my share of the work. We planned this on the trip home.
But on Monday, I felt well again. It was now the third day of being completely symptom-free. Free from pain, free from bleeding and I didn't have to go to the toilet as frequently. How can these major symptoms have disappeared so suddenly? And so completely?
I was curious. Had the kohlrabi played a part? Could I find out simply by eating more kohlrabi? So I drove to the supermarket and bought more kohlrabi. As of then, I had a raw kohlrabi every day. If supplies ran out, new ones were acquired. Luckily, kohlrabi is something that is always freshly available, almost everywhere.

Even over the following few days and weeks, I remained free from pain and any bleeding. I had no need for the heat cushions, had no pain, I could eat anything and could work. I felt well.

It was as if somebody had flipped a switch. What was happening to my body now? How was this possible? Could a raw kohlrabi heal an inflamed and severely weakened bowel? How could this be possible? Could it cure an autoimmune disease and stabilise an immune system? I was free, I was freed! I had got my body back and could sit at the table and eat again with my family, which I had been yearning for! I could go shopping, walk in the garden. Every day was a gift! Finally, I could put everything behind me. The pressure tailed off as did the anxiety and worry about the next day and those days still to come. At the weekends, I was now able to travel out to our plot of land where our house was being developed. The cellar was already complete, the children had laid beds in the garden and sown flowers and vegetables. They proudly showed me the success of their work. I was amazed and also planned to do something similar myself this summer.

At my next doctor's appointment, four weeks later, I explained enthusiastically to my gastroenterologist that I had been eating kohlrabi daily and since then had been symptom-free.
He listened to me attentively and studied me while doing so. I was extremely surprised by his response. He was of the opinion that the kohlrabi probably had nothing to do with my improvement and that it was more likely to be the medication that was now working; it had obviously just needed some time. Finally the time had come for them to have a positive effect. He was very pleased and said I should continue to do what I was doing and if I liked the kohlrabi then of course I could carry on eating it. As the saying goes: faith can move mountains. Maybe the doctor thought completely differently to me and thought I was a little eccentric. Perhaps he often had patients who talk about their "intuitions" and make quite crazy discoveries – that is, of course, not scientifically proven, and if it were so, then of course

science would have discovered it long ago, and he would know about it.

I found his remarks odd. I felt like he hadn't listened to me or we had been talking about completely different things. However, I had expected a completely different reaction, because I assumed that he would be interested, that he would take notes and maybe give this advice to other patients. I continually hear that the causes are not known, that the condition cannot be healed. Now I'm doing well but it appears that that is of no interest to anybody. Why?

He pushed the subject to one side to make room for the most important subject to him, my medication. At the end of the day, he's the doctor, not me. He has completed extensive education to become one. I can't simply walk in with a kohlrabi. Was my approach wrong? Did I take him by surprise? No. I'm the patient and I have gained profound experience and now feel symptom-free. However, I had hoped that my doctor would be able to explain it to me! What a success for him, he had healed me. For him, it was enough that the medication was working.

For me, that was the moment when I again started to view the role of some doctors involved in my treatment with a more critical eye.

The next few weeks were like a miracle because my skin problems also cleared up over the following months. The port-wine stain on my neck became increasingly paler, more and more often it would disappear for days at a time and after several weeks is was no longer visible at all. I slowly began to forget all about it.

I also had no hair loss, no weeping scalp eczema and no painful joints. My medication was 3x2 tablets of Salofalk daily and a kohlrabi.

Understandably, I was completely over the moon. A new life appeared on the horizon for me. I rejoiced in my newly restored health and enjoyed building our house. How easy so many things were all of a sudden.

Our house was extended by a second floor, it had a roof and had a clinker brick exterior, as is customary in Brandenburg. The garden was a huge building site and, when we had time, we pitched in. Since I was now feeling well, I could finally help out, especially because we were hoping to move into our house in the autumn.

Since I was healthy, renovating the house in which we would live, provided me with a lot of exercise. We had piles of books, about half of our removal volume was made up of books! So, I acquired some handy cardboard boxes from the office to store all the books temporarily in the basement of our office. This meant I could dismantle the bookshelves and paint each room, wall-by-wall, one after the other, while we were still living in the house. Physically this was absolutely no problem for me, it did me good. My girls also helped me a lot and the four floors were completely renovated by the time we were ready to move in. What a wonderful feeling to have a body filled with so much energy.

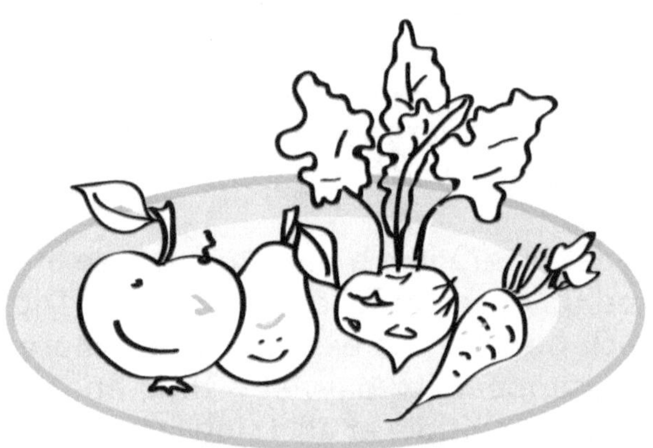

The work in the office continued of course, the order situation was good, building work costs money and I was fully involved. Our move took place at the end of August. We were very proud of what we had achieved! Despite the stresses of the last few months, I was doing so well that I had reduced the Salofalk in October to 3x1 tablets. I was still eating kohlrabi several times a week, but that was becoming increasingly less. I no longer took it so seriously. I was feeling very confident.

The arrival of the bill at the (year) end

I continued to tell different doctors and my circle of friends about my experience with kohlrabi; nobody could imagine that the healing of such a serious illness, for which so many medicines were necessary, could be possible by eating kohlrabi. I also think it sounds rather utopian now. Do you believe it? It's now been six months. I know it was like that but it really didn't matter to me because I felt cured and was floating on cloud nine because I was now no longer taking any medication.
At the end of November, I suddenly started again with some minor facial skin problems, and the port-wine stain reappeared. I was prescribed some of the Dermatop ointment, Leukichtyol and Remederm ointment for these symptoms but otherwise I felt very well. How could I have missed these signs? I was only eating kohlrabi now and then.

Our family was about to expand: the girls had wanted a dog for such a long time. In November, we were joined by our "Snoopy", a golden retriever, a dear friend, who both girls spoiled like a little brother.
The year came to an end. In the supermarkets, chocolate Father Christmases sparkled, seducing customers. The first Christmas holidays in the new house were approaching. It was such fun decorating the new house. It was wonderful that the year had ended on such a high note. I was healthy, our house was gradually getting finished. And I was really looking forward to the springtime so I could plan the garden.

On Boxing Day, we were invited to our friends' house, who we liked very much. Veronique is French and a fantastic cook! I enjoyed how lovingly she prepared everything and very much looked forward to the good food. It promised to be a wonderful evening.
However, by the afternoon I got a shock: I had blood in my stools. Had I eaten too much of the wrong things? Where had it come from all of a sudden? Had the good, substantial Christ-

mas dinner with roast goose played a role or the colourful plate of sweet treats? The evening that I had planned turned out to be very different for me. Helmut and the children drove to Berlin. I was no longer able to go; I wrapped myself in a warm blanket, had painful cramps that made me shake and so much gas in my stomach!
I still had enough Salofalk and increased the dose to 3x2 tablets. In my head, a world was collapsing, I was sad and alone that evening. Over the next few days, I slowly went downhill and I spent New Year feeling extremely worried. At the beginning of January, I had an appointment with my doctor.

Medication costs in 2000: 2036,80 Euro

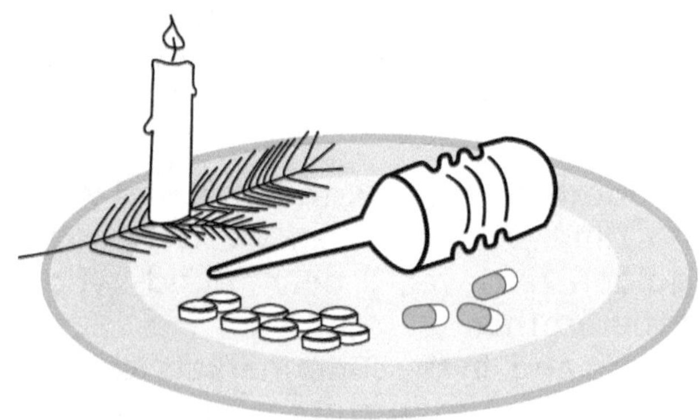

2001

And so it starts all over again

Why had I not immediately started to eat kohlrabi? That's what I ask myself now. I recalled thinking about it at the time but then pushing it to the back of my mind again! Why had I not trusted my own experiences? How could I have ignored them? Had I allowed myself to be influenced? It was so long ago. Had it irritated me that nobody had taken me and the kohlrabi seriously? Nobody had believed me so in the end I had doubted it too. Are we so fixated on "expert opinions"?
No doctor and no medication had been able to successfully treat my illness over the years. Those six months of eating daily kohlrabi had by far been my best time to date!

My doctor prescribed me Mutaflor®, Salofalk enemas and Salofalk tablets. On 8th February 2001, the health insurance company informed me that the costs for the Mutaflor® (intestinal bacteria) would no longer be covered with immediate effect because there would be no guarantee of a successful outcome. I desperately grabbed at every piece of information I could get my hands on. I received texts (MMW Advances in Medicine, Special Edition, C. Urban & Vogel Medien und Medizin Verlagsgesellschaft mbH 1999, When bacteria attack the intestinal wall, R. Duchmann, H. Loch and W. Kruis), which had detailed reports on the positive impact of intestinal bacteria in maintaining remission status.
In addition, the company Ardeypharm has written an Information leaflet on the use of Mutaflor® in human medicine: Effective principles and therapeutic safety of Mutaflor®. I found a lot of positive things in here. Medletters 3/99 from the Scientific Information Service. Ardeypharm describes a study: Ulcerative colitis – Mutaflor® and Mesalazine equivalent and there was also a supplement: Reimbursement of Mutaflor® in statutory and

private health insurance: essentially, only medications for the treatment of symptoms with pathological significance shall be reimbursed. This leaflet was from the manufacturer itself. So, did my symptoms have no pathological significance, or am I with the wrong health insurance company?

Thanks to this new cocktail of medication, I soon felt better again. But this remission phase in the February only lasted a few weeks. Again I tried to manage my professional life and push the illness to the back of my mind. The good thing was always that beforehand I had not known what to expect. At the beginning of April, another even more severe flare-up struck me. It affected my entire left colon and, in part, the transverse colon. I couldn't get my head around why my body was so hell-bent on destroying itself. Why didn't my immune system kick in at this point? Again I was prescribed Betnesol enemas.
So cortisone again, slept again, dozed here and there, torn away from life again, stopped in my tracks.
I asked to be prescribed magnesium for this because I already knew that the cramps in my legs would regularly flare up. Often the cramps just alternated and seemed to jump back and forth between my calf, foot, thigh and buttocks. They placed me in hopeless and very painful situations; my legs disobeyed me, and with my arms I fought helplessly.
In addition I was given vitamin E because, in the meantime, my joints had swollen up and were painful. And of course, I was also prescribed iron tablets.

I then moved into the basement of our new house, in a room with an embankment in front of the window so I had daylight. This meant that I wouldn't wake anyone with my restless sleep and night wanderings, or if I'm thrashing around and shaking during the cramps. The most important thing was the fact that I had my own toilet right next to me, JUST for me. What a luxury in my situation!
However, now I was imprisoned in the basement, I no longer managed to climb the stairs. My knee and elbow joints failed me. My body couldn't get up one single step on its own.

My children don't have many memories of my time in the basement. They came to see me after school, Fine would usually come down in the afternoons and Franzi often in the evenings. They were very kind, told me anything new that was going on at school, usually "well-wrapped in cotton wool" for mummy so as not to worry me and so that I didn't ask too many questions. I got a fresh, warm cup of tea and enjoyed having them spend a few minutes with me. It was wonderful to smell them, feel them and made me so happy to see how well they were and how full their day had been. Then they would go about their usual business: Fine would take Snoopy for a walk or go into her room to do her homework or play. I would usually fall asleep immediately thanks to the Betnesol. After her A-levels, Franziska did an apprenticeship as a system electronics technician at Siemens and didn't get home until late. When she was at home, the girls usually played and messed around together. It was often very funny, and the house was filled with the laughter of the children. Of course, there was the odd loud war of words but the air would soon settle once the storm had passed. I was really pleased with the children and it made me especially happy when they both came down to see me and sat on the edge of the bed, joking around. My biggest wish is that they will always stick to together throughout their lives and be there for one another. This thought occupies my mind often, it worries me that I am not able to be there often enough for them. When Helmut came home in the evenings, he would help me up the stairs so I could spend the evening together with my family, make myself tea and prepare the evening meal.

There's more

On 19th April, I had another appointment for a colonoscopy. During the course of the assessment, it was revealed that the effect of the cortisone had not been sufficient enough. A further increase in medication was required. As a result, the treatment was to be supplemented by immuno-suppressants. I was shocked at this prospect. Is my immune system, which is supposed to protect my body from illness, now going to be switched off by medication? I was not comfortable with this idea. What consequences would that have on the rest of my life? Up until now, I assumed my immune system was too weak, it had to be strengthened. Now it will be "shut down"! Was there no alternative? I discovered there wasn't. The immuno-suppressants would prevent my intestines from being damaged further. They would reduce the body's defence mechanism against my own immune system and as such prevent "self-destruction". They would also be effective against the recurring arthritis.

I would therefore have no immune system. How would that make me feel? What happens if I get a cold or an infection? Will I have to keep away from other people and animals or will I keep on getting new illnesses? Can you do without an immune system? I couldn't imagine the consequences, but I couldn't get any help either.

For the first time, I now had to come to terms with the fact that this would be a medication that I would probably have to take for the rest of my life. I had to now finally bury the hope that all this would stop at some point. I felt that I had to irretrievably say goodbye to a phase of my life, to the time of a carefree youth. Despite the prospect of the dose being reviewed after two years, my life was now probably dependent on medication forever. Blood tests were also necessary given the fact that I was taking Imurek. Initially at short intervals, then later at least once a quarter. An ultrasound of the liver, kidneys, pancreas and gall-bladder was carried out: liver normal, homogenous, bile ducts not blocked, no evidence of stones, pancreas and spleen unremarkable, kidneys o.k.

I had been taking the Imurek since May now. Medication starts slowly, with one tablet, and is increased to three tablets quarterly. Gradually my immune system will be released from its natural function. Then it should be firmly in the hands of the medication and the self-destruction of my body should finally stop.

Because it will take some time for the medication to reach the places that it is needed, I was to remain on the Betnesol enemas for a while longer, at least until this flare-up had subsided.
I was then signed off sick again. My only job was to: doze and sleep so that I could get better again. And of course my guilty conscience niggled at me because I was unable to do anything. Being a burden did not feel good. The severe flare-ups made me depressed. Or was it the medication? Am I going to need specialist nursing care soon? What's the next step? Will my family or my children have to look after me? Will I have to have bowel surgery? Will I then be given a stoma? But I am still so young and have so many plans. I have a wonderful family and an exciting job, my own company – I can't and don't want to imagine such a life. I am scared to be dependent and I fear my body's rapid decline because of this condition. Helmut always listened to me and often managed to make me laugh. He sees the positive. He must have a lot more to worry about than I do. Sometimes I fall into a feeling of despair, it's not good and it doesn't help anyone.
My daily medication: 1 tablet of Imurek, 3x3 tablets of Salofalk, 1x Betnesol enema, 3x1 Ferro Sanol, Magnesium, Moviprep. Weight: 51 kg.

Visit from the health insurance company

Also, during this time, I received a visit from the health insurance company. The representative initially went to the office to look for me. My employees explained that I was not in because I was ill. My health insurance company was naturally informed – otherwise it wouldn't have been there. The company knew both addresses as I had to specify them both. The insurance representative didn't announce his arrival. The next time, he came to the house. I could only be reached here if Helmut was still at home in the mornings. I was unable to get up the stairs alone. The Betnesol caused me to sleep far too deeply and I couldn't hear the doorbell in the basement. Helmut explained to the gentleman that I slept deeply, was rarely responsive during the day and sent him away. In addition to this, he explained that he would have to bring me upstairs therefore it would be wiser to make an appointment.

But who were these visits, every few weeks, supposed to be helping? There was an uneasy feeling that this was more a matter of control. I think that's what it should be called.

Some time later when I was feeling better, I invited him in to find out what he was after. He wanted to know whether everything possible was being done through my doctor to make me better, whether everything was going smoothly with the accounting at the insurance company and how long I thought that I would be ill for. I think this money could be invested better – for the patient -, especially since he could tell how I was feeling from my prescribed medication.

I have fond memories of not being not alone in the basement at this time. As soon as the last family member left the house early, our dog, Snoopy would come downstairs and lie next to me on the bed. When I was awake I would stroke him and chat to him. He would then lift his head up and look at me questioningly with his big brown eyes. When I had to go to the loo, he would follow me and wait patiently until I emerged again. It was comforting to spend time with him. He gave me warmth and peace thanks to his endless patience. He had time and was just there for me.

In the afternoons, Josefine would come home from school, Snoopy would hear her approaching the house and when the key turned in the lock, he would charge up the stairs, full of expectation. He knew, it was now time to go out! I was so happy always spending time with him and was thankful for the time that he had for me. I was also sorry that I couldn't take him for walks. In his loving devotion, he had become my fellow inmate in the basement.

After a few weeks, I felt better. The Betnesol had worked, or was it now the Imurek? Going up the stairs became easier each day and soon I was able to manage it alone again. Initially I left the house late in the evening or at a time when I knew that I was unlikely to bump into anyone. Fortunately, in the immediate vicinity, we had a large green field and of course, Snoopy was always more than willing to come with me, no matter how late it was. I would wear a long coat, which gave me the necessary security if I lost control. Because unfortunately, I couldn't just beam myself back to the house.

Our dog was still young and if he heard the word "walkies", he would jump around with excitement, he wanted to run and explore the world. He therefore had no understanding when my situation suddenly changed, if I had to turn around, even if we had only just left the house! He would then be completely confused by the world and in my distress, a fracas would break out. This would often make him pull strongly on his lead and worm his way out of his collar. Following his springtime emotions, he disappeared at full gallop into the distance. I just stood there – what was I supposed to I do? I had no choice. I could ONLY go back home. But how could a young dog be left to run around the town? I went home and called the office. Helmut drove back and around the town looking for him. Once I had got changed and felt more stable, I went to help him search. There was so much life in this fluffy little bundle! When we found him, he came over to me happily wagging his tail.

"I have missed you sooo much, where have you been?" Of course. When he came over like that, all my anger, anxiety and worry disappeared. "My darling, there you are, we have missed you so much, too!" He was wonderful, golden and sweet!

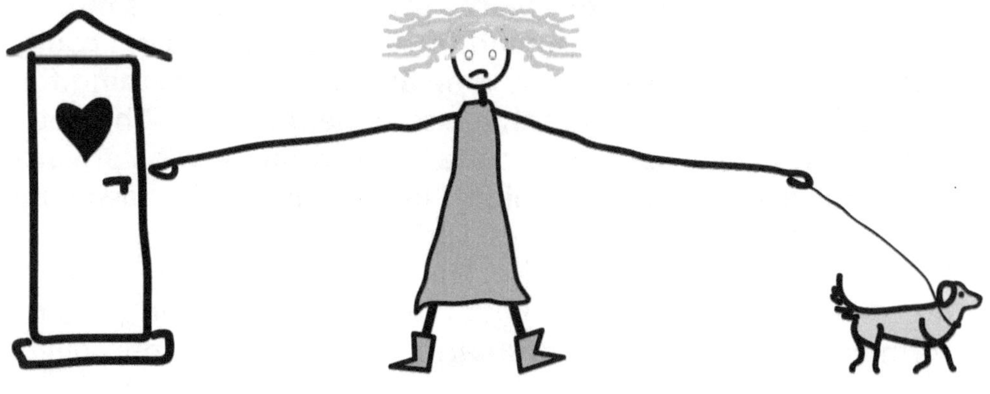

My condition slowly improved. I felt that regular exercise, and walking the dog, was good for me and stabilised me physically. These "trips out" made me feel like I had achieved something and like I had regained a piece of my life. It felt like a success and I was so happy about it. Every little success was motivation for the next step. It is important to keep getting up and carrying on.

To make matters worse, the port-wine stain now made an appearance on my neck. For a few weeks it was dark red in colour, then pink and for many months it was the first thing that greeted me when I looked in the mirror in the mornings. Like a thermometer, it displayed my current condition in colour.

Is the Imurek working?

In the spring, we laid out the garden around the house. I was in my element doing this. I knew how to design things. We had 40 cubic metres of garden soil delivered for the garden project. It was a huge mountain in the front garden and I had a job that would give me daily exercise in the fresh air. When I felt well, I took the rake and spread the soil evenly over the garden, gradually creating beds for vegetables, flowers, and a grassy area. I worked on it slowly and steadily as long as my strength would allow and felt really good doing it. I still didn't have enough strength to do any spade-work, however. When the children came home, they took the wheelbarrow and shovel and moved a few barrow-loads to the places I wanted them. This meant that I had enough soil to spread for the next few days. I could divide up my strength and my time and achieve something for my family. I now have a job that also benefits others. The path back to the house was often too far for me, but it was a private path, not exposed, so it wouldn't lead to any embarrassment like on public streets and places. Springtime was wonderful and I enjoyed the intensive exercise. The sun rose higher by the day, it got warmer and I noticed with horror that red pimples were forming on my torso and both arms. These quickly multiplied and in the end my arms had huge weals on them and were heavily swollen. It was a sun allergy. I obviously couldn't tolerate the sun anymore. So the Imurek had started to work. What was actually happening to my body this time? My doctor had NOT prepared me for this. I asked myself the question again. What are the outcomes if your own immune system no longer works? I didn't know. I discovered time and time again that on the doctor's bills, which I could check as a private patient, a consultancy fee was listed although that advice was something I was sorely lacking.

I called my dermatologist about the allergy. I got an appointment and explained to her that I was on my new medication, Imurek. For the sun allergy, I was prescribed Rp. Leuchkichthyol and Remederm Wiedmer cream. But it actually only helped me to avoid the sun and to cover my body accordingly.

It was this spring that Josefine had her "Jugendweihe" (coming-of-age party). This included a big celebration. What should I wear? I am a dress size EU 36 (UK 8) but for weeks I had been suffering from severe water retention in my legs. The choice in my wardrobe had been reduced to NOTHING because of it. Despite the happy occasion, I only had a dark black suit with an ankle-length skirt. Nor did I have any suitable footwear either because my feet had also swollen up. I was shocked by how extreme the water retention had become. I wasn't prepared for this side effect. Could this be blamed on the Imurek or on the combination of Imurek and cortisone? I had already got used to my thickened legs but it was only on this day that I had noticed that they had become so huge that I could barely put my hands around my ankles. I could no longer bear to look at myself in the mirror.

Over Whitsuntide, we travelled with friends to the Baltic Sea for a few days. The weather was just beautiful and we were really looking forward to the time away. Barely had we arrived, than we went to the beach to walk along the sea front. Very bravely we attempted to go into the water with bare feet and challenge the waves. The Baltic Sea is so wonderful. I actually don't want to spend a single year of my life without coming here. I find the sea has a relaxing and cleansing effect. I love the Baltic Sea, the sand, the expanse and the pure air.

After just one hour, the first red pimples started to show themselves again, my arms swelled and this time my neck and face were affected by it. I had hoped that applying the cream would have offered me a little more protection from the sun. I had also bought myself some sun cream with SPF 25 from the pharmacy. Wearing this sun cream, I looked as white as a snowman, but I was willing to do whatever helped! The weather was fantastic, the sky bright blue but I didn't have a chance! I went back to the holiday home alone and couldn't leave for the next three days. The weather was just too nice for me. The family could enjoy the time, I was pleased about that. They should be having a whale of a time and walking. That was some consolation.

By the end of July, the Imurek was increased by a further tablet, so now I was taking two tablets. Up until then however, it appeared to still not be having any effect on my bowel. I was going to the toilet less often but still had no control over my bowel from early morning through to the evenings. It took some effort for me to be able to leave the house and I was still in constant pain. I also felt exhausted and less resilient.

I was still supposed to take the cortisone daily until the end of August, and then slowly wean off it so long as I was still on sick leave.

I had high hopes of being more stable by then because the health insurance company hadn't accepted an extension since I was able to freely more around again and could go for walks several times a day. I sincerely hoped that the disease would gradually disappear through taking the Imurek, but at some point the medication had to work in the intestines as well!

I wanted to use the remaining time to get myself fit again and to be able to live well with the new medication despite the side effects. To do this, it was really important to me to bring an exercise and relaxation routine into my life. I reminded myself of the success I had with riding my bike and I wanted to pursue this again. If my bowel was calm by midday, I would go out on my bike. Snoopy could also accompany me on his lead. Unfortunately, this wasn't going to be possible if the weather was sunny because the warmer it was, the more I had to cover up. I also took the decision to do regular biofeedback for relaxation and balance to promote further healing.

Since I felt physically and mentally better, I deliberately came off sick leave. By doing this, I felt freer again in my decisions. From September, I was fit for work and I was very much looking forward it. I was back. Things could only get better now, so I hoped.

Coming back to the office after such a long time, it was astonishing to see how much had changed. Sometimes I felt like a stranger because I had to be told by my staff where things were kept. That was a new feeling for me. Before this, I was the one who had made the decisions and come up with ideas. I could do nothing but marvel at how much had happened and how Helmut had managed. Would I have been able to manage as well if it were him who had been ill?

I was very thankful to our staff for all their hard work. Nevertheless it was obvious that there hadn't been the time for certain things.

After just a few days however, it became evident that I needed an interim solution. It wasn't working. Frequently, I was unable to drive to the office because my bowel was too unstable. It was very unpleasant for me in front of the staff to not have it under control. I was embarrassed! Of course, I also had that feeling of "being dirty" and "smelling awful". I didn't want to keep on having to explain what was wrong because persistent bowel noises and uncontrollable flatulence were a constant stress that I didn't want to inflict on anybody.

It took an immense amount of energy to keep explaining, in response to friendly questions with a smile on my face, that I was doing ok. A few minutes later, I would be holding my tummy and running out of the room mid-conversation. I lacked the strength to work like this because I had to constantly pretend. The thought of being absent again for an uncertain amount of time caused me a lot of stress.

This is why we set up a working space at home. I actually deliberately didn't want a computer in the house because, in order to be able to really switch off after a long day of work, I wanted to have the time to myself. I found it relaxing to separate the office from home. Home was meant to signify the end of work! So for the time being, I only travelled to the office to make arrangements and time and again at weekends when I could look at, check and proofread all the work progress in peace. The pressure was so much less when I was at the office alone. I focused better and achieved more.

I hope that once the second tablet of Imurek had taken effect that the pain and bleeding would significantly regress, but the opposite happened.

As I read through the package insert, I discovered the following under the section on side effects: "Occasionally, in transplant patients, severe inflammatory diseases of the large intestine (colitis, diverticulitis) and intestinal rupture have occurred. In patients with inflammatory bowel disease, severe diarrhoea has been reported". I was very irritated. This medication was supposed to free me from colitis and diarrhoea?

My blood sugar

For some time now, I had had problems with my blood sugar. It struck me in particular on one Sunday when I was in the office. We were expecting visitors at home and I wanted to be back home for coffee-time in the afternoon. Some chocolate was lying on my table in the office, next to my computer (that was always important to me. I found sweet things to be a great source of energy to stay fit when I was stressed), but I thought, "Helmut has baked an apple strudel and it isn't far to the house". Once I had finished my work, I drove back home – on the way, the urge for something sweet was overwhelming. Just before I entered our village, my right arm began to shake, as if it had a life of its own. The left arm then started to move and was constantly in front of my face. I started to sweat profusely. I tried to control the right arm and in the process guide the steering wheel. I had to keep myself very together, I still had 3 kilometres ahead of me. I didn't understand what was happening to me in this moment. But I did know that I couldn't stop now as I needed sugar quickly! I parked up at the house, staggered out of the car and into the house and kitchen. I took the custard that had been prepared for the apple strudel from the cooker and some vanilla ice cream from the freezer. I stirred the ice cream into the custard, settled myself into a chair and with a HUGE SPOON stuffed THE WHOLE LOT into my mouth! I ate half a litre of custard in one go! I then felt much calmer. Our visitors hadn't arrived yet. Helmut must have just freshly made the custard.

I studied the package inserts of the Imurek and Betnesol again to check whether I had overlooked the fact that these drugs may hinder a person's driving ability, but there was nothing in there. Several times, I experienced something along similar lines and each time it really scared me. However, I had been warned and I wanted to use my bike more often to get to work anyway. But even that became a problem. Even the slightest effort led to a drop in my blood sugar, sweating and total weakness, accompanied by a strong feeling of dizziness. I had to dismount my bike and became fearful that my energy levels would not be enough for me to reach my destination.

Since he was 20, my younger brother had been diabetic. I was always really shocked when I saw how punctured his body was by the needles. Was I now getting this illness? What could I do to prevent something like this happening to me? Could the onset of diabetes be prevented? Who could give me advice on this? But, I didn't pursue the answers to these questions because I had assumed and hoped that once the cortisone was out of my system that the blood sugar problem would disappear again. I was also always convinced that if the Imurek was working then I would no longer need the cortisone.

In September I was prescribed a third Imurek tablet. Now my immune system should be under the complete control of this medication within the next few weeks. Would this mean that my body would have no more autoimmune reactions? Is it all over? Is my bowel now CALM? Will my joint pains stop too, especially in my hip joints and hands, which are also caused by an autoimmune disease?

I was now noticing changes in my skin on a daily basis. Small, superficial blood spots and small inflamed blood vessels were forming on my body, especially on my stomach area. I also discovered an increasing number of dark pigmentation spots, scattered warts, thickened veins, extensive broken blood vessels and spider veins. For the first time, I consciously witnessed how my body was ageing, really deteriorating. Almost daily, I observed negative changes.

Nobody had told me about the side effects of the immuno-suppressants before. I had not been made adequately aware of this nor given advice on preventative measures by my doctor nor was there anything in the package insert.

This medication made me feel disheartened and depressed. I could no longer remember how many weeks had passed since I last laughed.

How am I supposed to deal with these new observations? I had to watch myself quickly and visibly get older, how life was drawing to an end and I couldn't do a thing about it. I was still only 41 years old.

My bowel problems didn't improve in the slightest over the next few weeks. My immune system had disappeared, my autoimmune disease had remained. I still had no control over my bowel and was not free from pain. I was opening my bowels 20 to 35 times a day. My bowel reacted nervously: to weather, stress, food, heat, cold, the telephone – I had no idea what it didn't react to. It even reacted during the night, when I was sleeping or doing nothing. It couldn't go on like this. These constant failures were getting me down and I was becoming sadder and sadder. My future often appeared to me to be hopeless. Neither the doctor nor the health insurance company could provide me with a useful alternative. So, I had to search for the causes myself and find a cure. What had I not yet tried?

I searched helplessly for more information, read lots and tried all the tips from friends and relatives with great hope at finding some relief. I was disappointed time and time again! The laboriously cooked chicken soup, the warmed baby food in jars, boiled, puréed carrots, white bread with cheese, pumpernickel with honey, mashed potatoes with butter, crisp bread with herb curd, rice pudding with apple purée, probiotic yoghurt, multi-vitamin juices, malt beer, lecithin – nothing helped. A friend recommended that I eat salt sticks and another that I drink lots of cola. On that advice, I bought a whole crate of cola in litre bottles! I tried so many things indiscriminately, helplessly and mindlessly. Instinctively, I avoided fried foods. And followed the advice of the doctors to avoid raw vegetables so that the in-testinal walls had to do less work and did not become any more damaged. I was particularly advised to steer clear of fibre-rich foods by all parties spouting scary prophecies: the peels and the seeds of tomatoes, gherkins and kiwis could hang around in the intestine, fresh strawberries were also not recommended be-cause of their fine seeds. The peel of raw apples, apple cores, nuts – everything could lead to inflammation of the intestines because it could get stuck somewhere. I also had to take into consideration the possibility of the intestines rupturing!

I searched for a nutritionist. She advised me to avoid all grain products, to boil everything, to eat a lot of soft boiled vegeta-bles and lean meat and a lot of fish. In addition, I should drink three litres of water a day. She also recommended mineral sup-plements. I saved myself the cost of another session. I had al-ready tried all those things! All this well-meaning advice from everyone was confusing my mind.

I read some time ago that microwaves are said to be harmful to health because they are not sufficiently shielded from their radiation, mostly to the outside. Is that supposed to happen? I tried it and put my mobile phone inside it. It rang loudly when I called it. The microwave has been in our kitchen all these years. We used it regularly to warm up meals and drinks. It was a mod-ern-day work facilitator but what effects was this radiation hav-ing on my body, if I already react to telephones? Using it couldn't be healthy in the long run. So, bye bye, microwave!

I also viewed pans coated with Teflon with a critical eye. In order to not damage the coating, you were supposed to use a wooden spoon. I did this consistently, nevertheless, after some time the coating still wore off. So where was it going? How much of it had gone into our meals? The coating contains benzene (which is incidentally contained in many soft drinks and flavoured waters). Since aluminium is also a harmful toxin, we bought stainless steel pans.

Since I first started working, I have drunk coffee early in the morning. My blood pressure had always been low and this helped me. Nevertheless, I completely gave up coffee now, because I noticed that it had an unpleasant effect on my bowel movements. I now drink green tea and I feel that it stimulates the intestine less. And my headaches are still under control.

What can help me? What do I need? Vitamin supplements? I took vitamin E. I also regularly took magnesium tablets for the ever-increasing cramps. I drank stomach and bowel-friendly teas. What else could I do? I had no more ideas left? At the end of the day, I never knew whether the pain was a direct consequence of what I had just eaten or a result of the last or next to last meal or the meal from the previous day? Or was it a result of a confluence of different things in the intestines? Maybe I should just keep eating the same thing so that I can find out? Who can give me trustworthy advice on nutritional issues? The doctors haven't been able to so far.
What role does my no-longer-existing immune system actually play in the digestion of foods? Can it still protect me against foreign bodies/toxins? I didn't know anything about this!
I tried to limit myself to a few foods and, similar to the way I used to cook purées for my children, I now prepared my food: boiled carrots with egg yolk, potatoes with butter, pasta with scrambled egg. Why does the stomach bloat with such simple dishes? Why is it now burning like acid? Why is it just blood and then watery diarrhoea again? I couldn't see the logic in it.
So, I thought about writing down and comparing everything I ate over the days. A big problem here was that I didn't eat any proper meals. I intuitively grabbed something to eat when I felt like my bowel was calmer and more relaxed – and of course I had to eat something. Since I wanted to put weight on, I used sugar. But I felt that my bowel didn't like this. It would grumble

more than usual. Ice cream and sweet desserts that I would indulge in to feed myself up usually led to problems immediately after eating, even though the food had not yet arrived in the gut! I got the impression that the burning sensation in particular was triggered by eating too many sweet treats. I assumed that I needed sugar to stop me being so cold, to gain more energy, to put a little weight on but obviously it didn't happen that way for me. What kind of energy-rich food is available? Is there really no other support? Is there no international research other than the same old dietary recommendations that are not remotely helpful for me?

All the nutritional recommendations from my doctors have so far not brought the slightest improvement; in some cases even the opposite. The recommended special foods were rusk biscuits, white bread, lean sausage paste or cooked sausage and cheese even seemed to trigger the burning. And sometimes what helped today, didn't help at all the next day. Even my cooked vegetable purées, soups or meat broths rushed through me like a flash flood and cause me a lot of pain!

In September the illness worsened, a new flare-up was approaching and I was prescribed the Betnesol enemas again. It was clear to me now that even taking the full dose of Imurek was affecting my immune system but not the colitis. It really bothered me now that I had to use cortisone again despite the strong medication. There was no getting around it since the pain was unbearable. I had really hoped that the subject of cortisone would be over forever now because my biggest fear was that I would have problems with my blood sugar again and there was a real risk of me becoming diabetic.

Why are there always only exit routes that make things worse? Why was my life becoming more and more difficult? But nothing helped, as hard as it was for me, first I had to go through these weeks taking the Betnesol, because I wanted to stop the acute progression of the disease, then I hoped to be able to reduce the dose slowly but quickly.

How can things go on like this? Was there really no end to the misery? Despite the constantly negative experiences with medication – because the effect did not last long – initially each new medication always gave me a glimmer of hope that my body, with this new help, would be able to stabilise itself again, perhaps even for the long term.

Ulcerative colitis –
a diet-related Western disease

At the end of October, we were invited to a birthday party at a friend's house in the village. I knew that the host, Lonny, was a very good cook and noticed that she only used specially selected ingredients that she bought at health food shops. She had often told me about this. These things were all completely new to me. I found it all very interesting but very time-consuming and as such completely unrealistic for me. She cooked in a different, healthier way, because it made her feel much better. When she went shopping, she grumbled about lots of things in the gro-cery stores that I had never really been concerned about, that I hadn't even noticed before. However, since we weren't going to be the only guests at the party, I had to cancel the visit. But Lonny was persistent and spoke to Helmut, who then begged me to come along, adding that she had some important infor-mation for me. She promised that there would be something that I could eat at her house, something that I would most cer-tainly would be able to tolerate! And that she would be really happy to see me!
The decision wasn't easy for me but I couldn't refuse Helmut's request! I didn't have to eat much, and if necessary I could go home. It wasn't far and Helmut would drive me! I was now re-ally pleased to have been invited, even more so by a lady who tolerated my problems and understood me and my concerns. It was a good feeling and I was finally happy that getting out of the house had been made so much easier for me. It was to be a very important evening for me, but I didn't know that at this early stage.

So, off we drove to the birthday celebrations. Lonny said to me: "I've found something in one of my books which I'm sure you'll be interested in. Can you believe it? It mentions your illness." More importantly, it states there that this disease can even be cured by eating a proper diet. "Look here, your disease is called ulcerative colitis", and she showed me a book with the following text:

"… decades of observations in clinic and practice have led me to the conclusion that ulcerative colitis and Crohn's disease are diet-related Western diseases that with consistent, strict dietary measures can even be cured. However these measures must be carried out over a very long period of time – in severe cases for years – and under very strict conditions. The best healing foods are clean, fresh foods.

It went on:
A standard diet weakens the general power of resistance, exacerbates the progression of the disease and hampers healing. …"

from: *Liver, Gall bladder, Gastro-intestinal and Pancreatic Diseases, Dr. med. M. O. Bruker, 19th edition, 2001, Page 162 ff.*

This was incredible information. How was this possible? This book was not new. What was written in it sounded very convincing to me, especially since it corresponded to many experiences. Why had I not already considered this myself? I took the book home to read. I wanted to try it now.
Lonny showed me her grain mill which she used to mill a small amount of grain every day for herself and her husband. The milled grains were then soaked overnight and covered with a plate. It all looked like a grey, sticky mass – not very appetising and I wondered how long I would be able to endure something like that. Lonny told me that she had been eating like this for years; the addition of fruit makes it all much tastier

You are what you eat

This evening changed so much in my life, especially my attitude to food. However, I had a long way to go. I remembered reading something similarly "confusing" as in this book, and it was in fact in a patient information leaflet from the company, Alfred-Nissle. I also thought back to the time when I had eaten kohlrabi every day.

The next day I read the book again and was amazed at the importance of nutrition in many other diseases. The connections were clear to see. "Dietary problems exist because we have moved too far away from our natural nutrition. We believe the advertising and the industry more than our natural instincts", writes Dr. Bruker. He also says, that diseases usually take decades before they break out. So we don't notice them until it's too late. It is essential to find the causes of a disease, I read, and that these causes have a lot to do with us and our lives. If I manage to change my life, and thus myself, will that have an influence on my illness? If it's down to me, I can do this!

Paths are made by walking them.

Franz Kafka

I will just make a start. I have nothing to lose. I will transform my diet and change my lifestyle. But where do I start? Where do I get the necessary information from? The more I thought about it, the more questions I asked myself. What does natural mean? Where can I get good quality wholemeal bread from? Which foods in my cupboards can I still use? What can I buy where? And what recipes can I use? I didn't know the answers to many questions yet.

How do I make this fresh porridge? I felt hungry and had no idea how to begin! As if she had read my mind, Lonny was suddenly standing at the door. She brought me her travel hand mill, which she didn't need at the moment and asked whether I needed anything as she was going shopping in Berlin. My face probably looked like one huge question mark because that was one of the questions currently going through my mind. "Do you have any grain?", she asked. No, I didn't have any. Where do I even get it from? Grain has never been on my shopping list before. She just laughed and said she would bring me everything that I needed. Back then, I didn't even know where to go to buy grain! Today, twelve years later, grain is one of my weekly purchases, and it is now also available in some supermarkets.

In the afternoon the bell rang again, and Lonny was standing in front of the door with a big basket full of brown paper bags, back from shopping in Berlin. The basket was huge! The contents were heavy! I was speechless and looked through it all curiously. The bags were labelled and contained different kinds of grain: rye, wheat, spelt, oats, barley and buckwheat. There were also sunflower seeds, linseeds and nuts. I had heard of the grains from my childhood local history classes, but how to make something tasty and healthy from them was still a mystery to me.

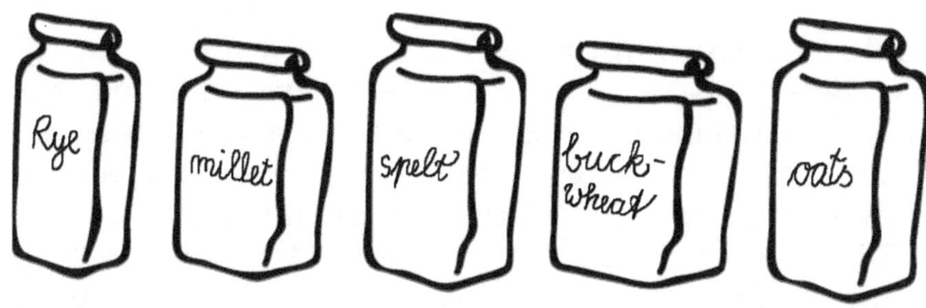

My first fresh grain dish

I remembered the recipe from the Bruker book. It talked about milled grain. It was a good thing that Lonny had lent me her hand mill, I could now give it a try. At first glance, it looked like a pepper mill. You could fill it using a small spoon. I poured a mixture of spelt and oats in and began to grind! It took time for the three tablespoons of grain to reappear as flour in a small glass bowl. This was my first self-ground wholemeal flour. The smell of the freshly ground grain reminded me of my childhood days in my grandfather's mill. Mixed with some tap water into a porridge, the ground grain should be left to swell for a few hours according to the recipe, and in this consistency it should be easier for my body to break it down. I had taken the first step on my new path. I was proud of myself.

Two hours later, I saw the result. Grey and sticky, not very appetising at first glance. I tried some of it. It was soft, tasted slightly nutty and was not as bland as I had feared.
According to the recipe, an unpeeled, grated apple with some lemon juice should now be added to it. I did that and the porridge was fluffier and much more aesthetically-pleasing. Next, I chopped up a banana into small pieces and stirred it in, the whole thing was now creamier. I now had the basis for a fresh grain dish. The recipe recommended the fruit of the season as a complement and for decoration. My fridge and basement provided me with pears and grapes. Sliced, with small blobs of whipped cream and decorated with walnuts, I now had a considerable treat in front of me! Although I was really hungry, from experience I ate it slowly and carefully – it tasted amazing! My stomach indicated a feeling of pleasure and satisfaction. Even after an hour, all was calm in my bowel and I felt well. My gaze wandered again to the baskets filled with all those bags. That is quite a different approach, I thought. I was now sure that I could do this since there was no trace of a burning feeling in my gut. Also in the course of the evening I had a clearly more pleasant gut feeling, I felt better, I felt more balanced. Is it possible that I could feel well after eating?
I still slept in the basement, I was finishing the cortisone this week. I was careful, unsure but nevertheless I somehow felt content. I want to hold on to this opportunity, cherish and nurture it. If you can really alleviate this disease in this way, then I'll learn everything, no matter how complicated the change is or how different the recipes are, at least that's what I had in mind for the time being.

That night, I slept well. And my first thought in the morning was that I could have this meal again today! I'll be using this hand mill every day, that's for sure. I was very thin and I felt weak after almost overcoming the flare-up. Some time ago, Helmut had put a comfortable rocking chair in the kitchen for me, from there I had the perfect view of the lively hustle and bustle of my family. So I sat in my chair, turned the mill and enjoyed the full and satisfied calmness in my tummy. The pain on this day was considerably less than the previous day.
Each day, my family watched my "milling" with amusement. What a wonderful mum! Maybe it would be good for them too. I had to put up with a few jokes here and there.
But it take long before my family wanted to try it too – it looked decidedly tasty because I really indulged myself! What's a crumbly bread roll with liver sausage or Nutella compared to a bowl of fluffy, aromatic and colourful breakfast served with fresh strawberries, blueberries, cream and nuts?

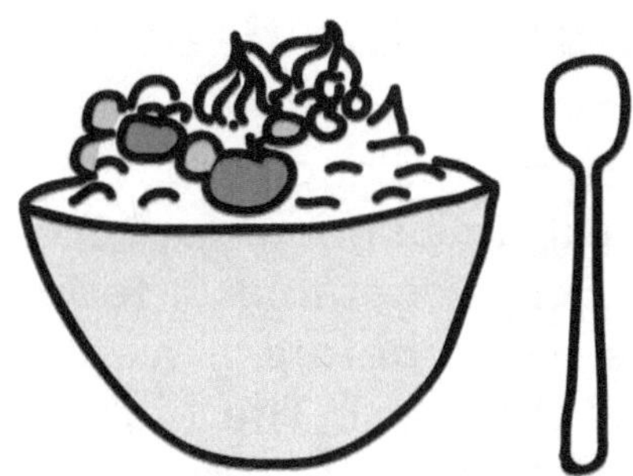

Healthy cooking sounds daunting and restrictive to many people. Just looking into a bag of grain required a lot of imagination. The fresh grain dish tasted better to me than anything I had ever tasted before for breakfast. Of course, I was happy to pass my bowl around now! Everyone immediately noticed that this dish not only looked impressive but also tasted fantastic. After a few days, I was now having to grind grains for four people every day – and that was some work with only a travel hand mill! Once again, we were all eating a family breakfast together; a grain-based, fruit salad. Both girls lovingly christened the dish "mud punch", my grandchildren now call it a "knight's meal", and Snoopy didn't care what the name was, he just saw the large bowl on the table and waited longingly every day in the hope of getting something out of it. He loved this dish too. It did me good being able to participate in family life in this way. I could do something for my loved ones again and it was also good for my soul.

It was amazing for me that the pleasant feeling of satiety lasted for several hours after eating the fresh grain dish. I felt no hunger, and I felt that my body was sufficiently supplied with energy. It was not only this relaxed feeling, but also a feeling of pleasure and joie de vivre, which had now returned. My mood was improving daily and everyone appeared to notice it. With this fresh grain dish, I had taken the first step towards turning my diet around. It consisted of 100% raw, fresh ingredients. So I was having ONE wholesome, raw food meal each day. But what do I eat next?

Raw foods – the path to healing?

The fresh grain dish did me good, but what do I do next? What should I eat the next time I'm hungry? So I took the next step. Since I've always liked vegetables, I found it easy. Raw foods should always be eaten before a warm meal and form the largest portion of the meal. The higher the portion of raw foods, the greater the chance of successful treatment. Raw food is healing food, wrote Dr. Bruker.

"An apple a day keeps the doctor away". I have always loved eating apples. Even now, I can still remember how special the apple harvest at a friend's house was for me and my siblings as children. Our city apartment would smell of apples in the run-up to Christmas. Each of us would lock away the biggest and most beautiful specimens from our excursion in our writing desks as if they were gold treasure. As part of my packed lunch, I had an apple every day throughout my entire school life. But can I just eat a raw apple now, if my intestines are still inflamed? The scheduled cortisone intake was only planned for the current week.

My stools were thin, my intestines very painful, I was opening my bowels more than 30 times a day. Will this not lead to a new flare-up? Wasn't it all a little too soon and too fast?

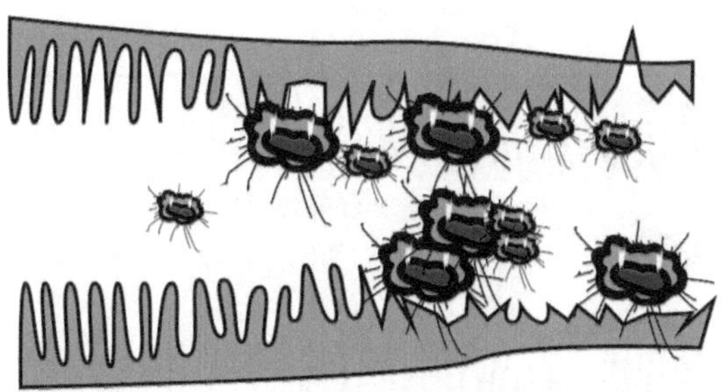

There was raw apple in the fresh grain dish. And I had tolerated it very well! So I ate an apple and a kohlrabi, which I already knew I could tolerate during a period of inflammation. I ate very slowly, chewed very thoroughly and was full afterwards. That was easy. I didn't get the impression that the fibres of the raw foods caused me problems in this condition. Chewing thoroughly (30 to 40 times) best prepares the food for the stomach. The enzymes can work and the high fibre content was good for my bowel. It also made my stools soft which prevented any constipation pains. Today, I know that our intestinal flora consists predominantly of bacteria, fungi and yeasts. The role of the bacteria is to more or less completely break down the remaining indigestible fibres (polysaccharides = multiple sugars) for the small intestine. The body, especially the human intestine, therefore needs time to adjust to this new diet. After antibiotic treatment, the microbiota of the intestine also has to be regenerated. The bowel is a very special organ because it has its own brain, the enteric nervous system. This includes a gigantic microbiome made up of millions of micro-organisms, not all of which have been researched yet. 90 per cent of these cells are intestinal bacteria, only 10 per cent belong directly to our bodies. They form a perfectly functioning system that not only breaks down our food but also produces important active substances such as vitamins and hormones! This also includes the body's own anti-depressant, serotonin. Maybe that's why I "hit rock bottom" so often when the disease was active? Our digestion is a very complex process and a change in all dietary habits takes time. You could think of it this way: dietary fibres mean full employment for our intestines, which in turn is good for our immune system.

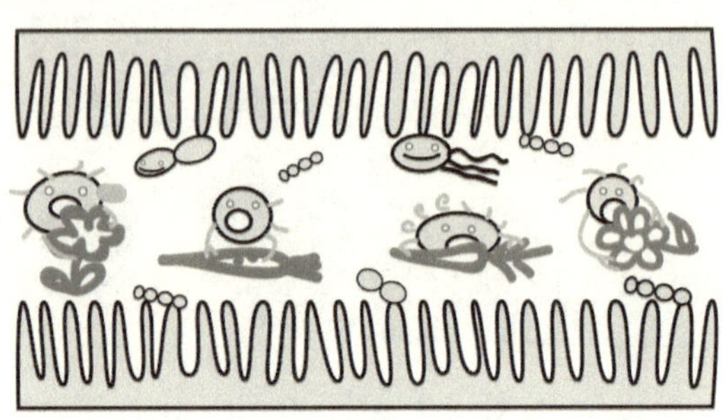

So I began with selected products which I knew would do me good. FOR ME, kohlrabi, carrots and apples were just like the fresh grain dish. They made me feel better every day. If I felt that it would do me good, I would add it to my daily menu: gherkins, radishes, black salsify, turnips, peppers, tomatoes and green salads.
I cut the colourful vegetables into pieces or prepared them as a salad. To start with, I usually decided on a colourful vegetable platter with chopped vegetables. I would also add sour cream with herbs, sea salt and garlic for dipping. I ate enough of the vegetables until I was full. I didn't notice a single problem. I must add that I didn't eat anything else at first. I didn't drink milk, didn't eat bread, had no sugar, no coffee – and besides apples, I ate no sweet fruit. I listened to myself, observed my body. Since I was doing so well, I added more vegetables to my platter and a variety of fruit: corn, celery, leeks, radishes, pears and bananas. My lunchtime dish was becoming increasingly colourful and I was improving by the day!
After four weeks, I was astonished at how much had already changed. The number of times I was opening my bowels had reduced by half and I hadn't felt so well in such a long time, since the pain had also reduced.

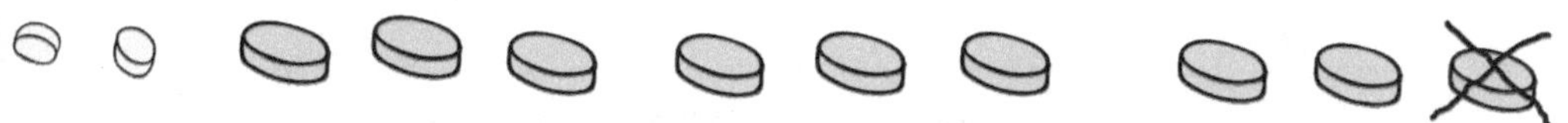

For this reason, I decided to take one tablet less of the Salofalk (of 3x3 daily tablets). This wasn't overconfidence, it was my good and relaxed gut feeling that was giving me this advice. However, the unexpected reaction came immediately. The next day, I opened my bowels five more times and had noticeably more pain! I then prescribed myself half a day of bed rest and biofeedback. I was very surprised at the direct effect of the Salofalk. I often felt that it wasn't having any impact and didn't seem to be working. I was now trembling and hoped that it hadn't triggered a new flare-up and everything I had done had been in vain! The next day, I had three less bowel movements and the pain decreased again. I actually counted my daily bowel movements because otherwise I wouldn't have believed it myself! On the second day, I felt better still. Could this be due to the reduction of just one single tablet? I was astounded by this effect. It showed me that the medication was having an effect. But it also confirmed that this nutrition was having some success too! This knowledge made me happy and content.

I was still very thin and was always cold. It's a general phenomenon with me that I feel even colder after every meal. My big worry at the beginning was that I would become thinner and thinner because of the raw food diet.

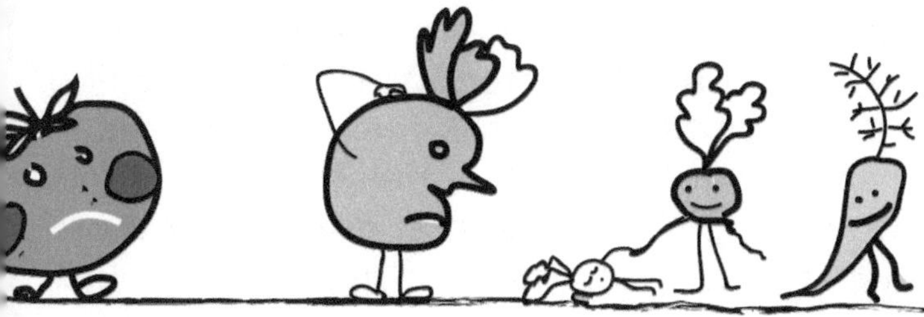

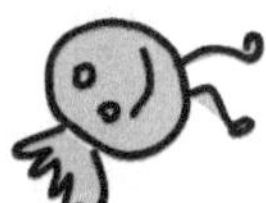

But with cream please!

It was December, I was almost exclusively eating raw foods. The very thought of it often made me shiver. At first I ignored it because to me there were no alternatives and I didn't want to take any risks. I tackled the change in diet slowly because I wanted to see how well I tolerated each foodstuff before adding it to my ingredients. Of course, it also wasn't easy to cook for the family at the same time. I had to get into a routine. To warm myself up, I drank a hot tea after dinner. The most important thing now was to start, and to do so with just a few, manageable things. Gradually, this would be increased so I took comfort during this time.

Of course, I kept myself informed about whole foods. At first glance, cream is a contradiction to a healthy diet. But I learnt something here too. Cream in a fresh grain dish provides our bodies with important fat-soluble vitamins. Cream is also a wonderful flavour enhancer. According to the recipe, you can add two tablespoons of this delicious treat per person to the fresh grain dish. However, I read that I can add as much cream as I like. Ultimately, fruit and vegetables contain no fat and I'm eating nothing else throughout the whole day! So, I spoilt myself with cream on a daily basis.
However, I did only eat organic whipping cream as it doesn't contain the additive carrageenan. Carrageenan ensures that the cream doesn't separate. It is also produced from red algae, is indigestible and is suspected to irritate the intestinal mucosa.

After two more weeks, my condition had noticeably improved again. I continued to count my daily bowel movements and also to clearly record the decreasing pain intensity. The fear of going to the toilet decreased significantly. I was feeling brave again and omitted another tablet of Salofalk. It had the same effect as before! More bowel movements and consequently more pain. Just three days later, everything settled again! This could-

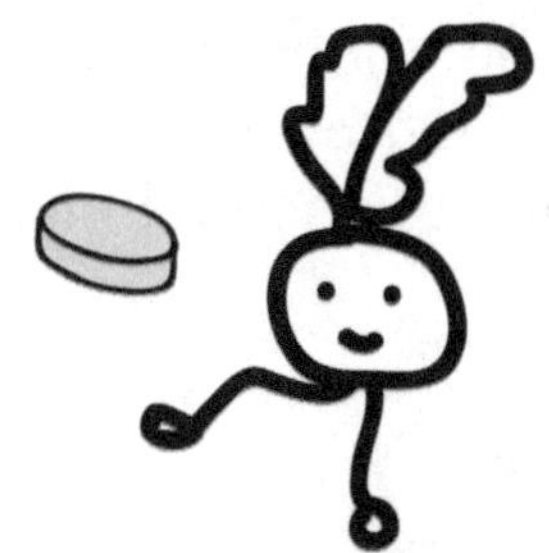

n't be a coincidence, I thought. However, I wasn't completely sure. How could this be possible? But at the same time I felt euphoric!

Initially, I was very strict with myself, I ate raw foods almost exclusively. My body got used to this during this time. The high fibre content in the raw foods filled me up for a long time. Three meals a day was sufficient. Cooked food only played a small role in the first few weeks of my dietary transition. So I can say that for me the raw food actually was a crucial turning point in my health. I wondered whether I could perhaps live on less medication in the future. It was a dream, yet it seemed more realistic by the day.

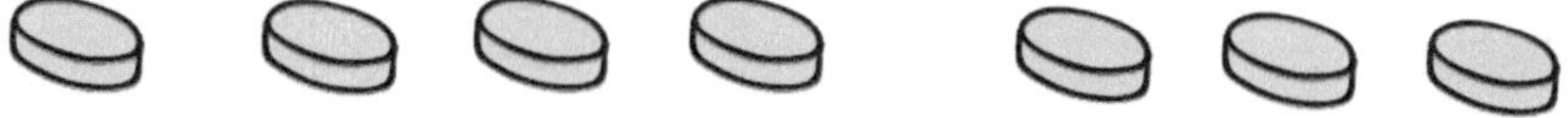

The next two weeks also brought further stability, the number of daily toilet visits sank, the pain decreased and I felt better. I reduced the Salofalk. And again, I had the same relapse!
I became happier and more relaxed, I felt as if my energy was returning. Both the pain and the number of bowel movements reduced noticeably by the day. It produced in me a whole new attitude towards life. All of a sudden, I regained my confidence to do many things again because I felt the improvements as each day went by! Less bowel movements, less pain, more confidence and, with it, more life! It was a fascinating time for me and an incredibly powerful experience. I could now go to the toilet feeling calmer and more relaxed. I no longer had to run. Once again I felt my entire body and not just my intestines. Until

then going to the toilet had been a cramping experience, now it had become a relieving one. Maybe only someone who has experienced similar things can understand this!

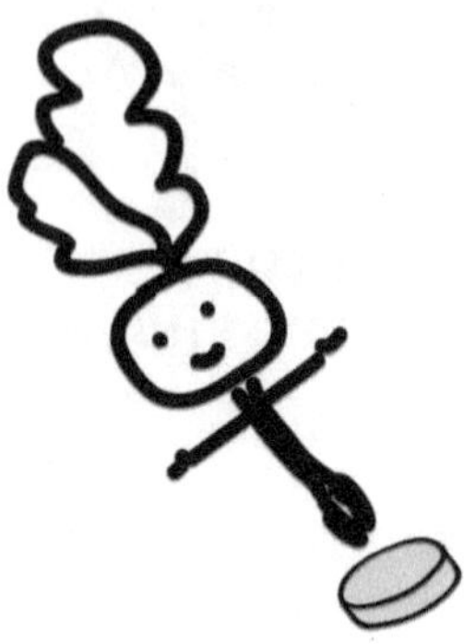

I had now omitted three Salofalk tablets; I started changing my diet two months ago. Through these experiences, I was gaining more and more confidence in this form of nutrition. My self-confidence grew with the reduction in medication. I felt that each day something negative was falling away from my shoulders. It wasn't the same feeling that I had after taking the cortisone and the subsequent improvements. It was a feeling of happiness coupled with an increase in strength and courage to face life.

I was once again enjoying time with my family and in my head I had more and more ideas of what I wanted to do. As well as my good mood, the fresh grain dish had had an effect on me from the very first day that Dr. Bruker had failed to mention: I was in the mood for physical love again, and at an intensity that showed I had a full six years to make up for it! Of course, Helmut was not remotely upset by this; there were days though when it was the afternoon before he arrived at the office. The staff had limited understanding because we were – given the

circumstances – not contactable by telephone. Helmut had a sunny disposition. He was no worse off than I was. We were just happy about it!
The last two months had been very good for me. I didn't think anything could go wrong anymore.

Medication costs in 2001: 3396,61 Euro

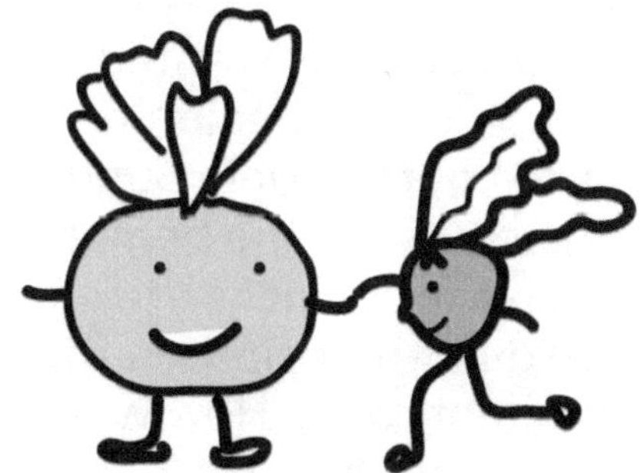

The long road to healing

2002

A new attitude to life

What will this year bring me? Will I be able to reduce my medication further? Maybe I will even defeat this illness? I was still very thin, 53 kilograms and I really wanted to put some weight on. However, I felt well! Since the beginning of January, we had been attending a dance course; every Sunday at 6pm. When I enrolled us both on the course at the beginning of December, I had only changed my diet four weeks previously. Another four weeks before that, I had been dozing on the Betnesol enemas despairingly in my basement room. How was this possible? I was all of a sudden doing things that had been unimaginable for me for years, that no longer just took place in my dreams and that I appeared to have completely lost: I voluntarily left the house, I had fixed deadlines and enjoyed being with people! And it was for these things that I now had an irrepressible desire! I was back in real life, and I'd fought for it myself. And now I had a lot of catching up to do!
I still remember that at the beginning, during the dance lessons, I always had my eyes on the toilet and had to visit it several times during the breaks. It wasn't that I couldn't get through the class or that I had to overcome the journey there, I could control it to a large extent.

The result of the change in diet to predominantly raw food meant that everything had to be rearranged in my tummy. At first it bubbled and rumbled constantly but my body, the bacteria in my intestines, adjusted itself to this diet. I had to give it enough time and tolerate these problems.

In our bowels, there are bacteria, yeasts and fungi, which work for us and for which we provide the ideal living environment. With an entire mass of around two kilograms, the micro-organisms weigh significantly more than our brains. In our daily diet, we all determine which strains feel at home in our bodies, which we invite in and which have to go.

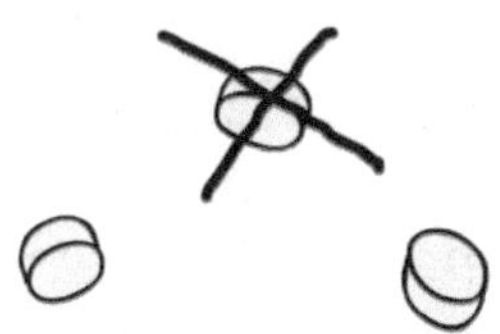

Golden Marie

It was the beginning of February. I had started to change my diet three months previously. My health was improving daily. I could not in any way have imagined the extent of this current success. I felt that I was being constantly blessed with luck. I felt like Golden Marie in the Brothers Grimm fairytale, Mother Hulda. So I decided to remove one of the Imurek tablets. I didn't want to consult a doctor about it because I had nobody in whom I could trust, nobody who I felt understood me. And of course, it had to be a doctor, who was well versed in nutrition and diet! I was sure that I could take the responsibility myself for this decision because I felt vindicated on a daily basis! And then I thought to myself: when I started the Imurek, I had no other information to hand. Nobody had explained to me what was happening to my body and what I could expect in detail. Now I am simply turning the use of medication around. I wanted to get my body back bit by bit. If I feel well, I will drop off one tablet every three months.
From now on I would take only 2x Imurek and 3x2 Salofalk tablets. I was aware that I wouldn't feel an immediate effect, and that the reduction in immunosuppressants would not be felt until the next quarter. But I had a good gut feeling about it.

A new spring

I continued to enjoy the daily improvements. I recorded these changes very accurately and my stomach then made the decision to reduce the medication again. In February and then again in March, I omitted another Salofalk tablet. Five to seven bowel movements a day, predominantly in the mornings, made my daily life so much more relaxed. The setbacks after dropping a tablet were significantly less but still noticeable, and after two days everything was good again. These reactions no longer shocked me. I knew it would only be for a short time and that it would always happen! For me, these experiences were reliable and I was convinced that my health progress was a result of my changed nutrition. This increased my confidence in my own body immensely.

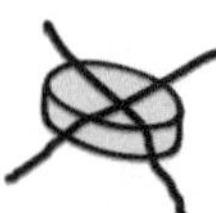

Following on from the raw foods, I tried small portions of warm meals. What I ate often came from the family kitchen. Warm vegetables for example were not a problem, also jacket potatoes, wholemeal rice and wholemeal pasta were more and more often a feature on the family dinner table Everyone was getting more and more used to wholemeal cuisine every day, which made it so much easier for me. Nobody had to! And Helmut often cooked something different for the children to fulfil their

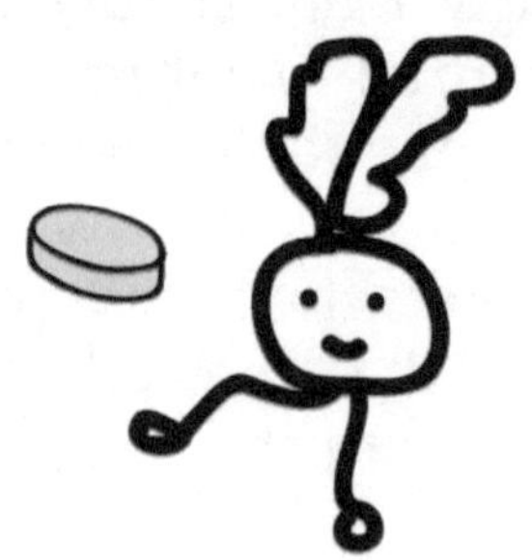

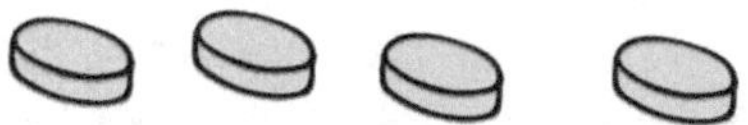

wishes. I changed our cooking habits by using only fresh vegetables (no tinned food), everything only al dente, so firm to
the bite, and cooked in a little water. The vegetable water was
reused or drunk. I add butter on the plate first so as not to heat
it. It tasted good and became more normal every day. Since I
couldn't identify any negative physical reaction after reducing
the first Imurek tablet, I became braver and dropped the second
tablet after another three months, in April. So I was now only
taking 4x Salofalk and 1x Imurek daily. I had also gained a further two kilos in the last few weeks.

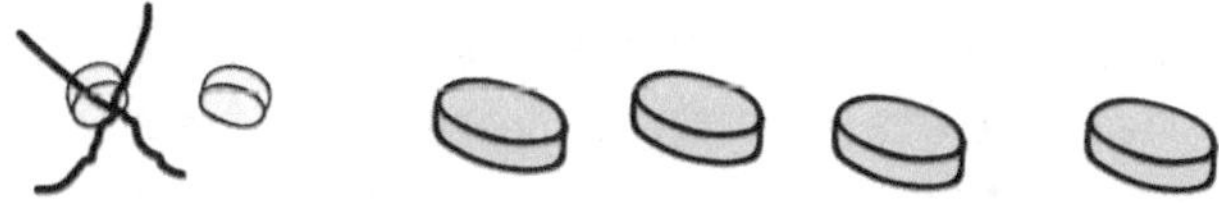

I was so grateful to my family for putting up with everything
and giving me the space to make these changes. I felt that I had
achieved so much for myself and for us in doing so.

Springtime inspired me: I got a craving for my old hobby from
my younger days and I started to paint again. I had freely available time now that I had regained my health. The children were
bigger and didn't constantly need me around. So I took my
paper, pencil and a folding seat and set off. I painted in nature
or in the village and each time I took myself further away from
the house. Only ever as far as I felt comfortable! And it always
went well. I was also pleased with my first sketch and all these
positive experiences took away more and more of the uncer-
tainty of the last few years.
I felt so much joy in painting again that I decided to look for a
group. Near to my office, a new adult evening class had just
started, ideal for newcomers.

I was enthusiastic about it and, in May, I planned to set up my own art group in the village. So I placed an ad in the local gazette and hoped for a great response. The interest was immense and lots of people told me how they had been waiting for such an opportunity. Where had I got the strength and courage for these activities from?

Warm dishes

I am now more and more occupied with preparing nutritious hot meals. I find that warm dishes caress my soul. Initially I found simple cream of vegetable soups very beneficial because after a large plate of salad, I always needed something to warm me up. Since I had completely given up tinned foods, I had the seasonal vegetables that were on offer in the supermarket. I discovered that there was a large range that I had never used in a soup before. Including celery, red beets, parsley roots, parsnips, red cabbage, peas, courgettes, sorrel, radishes, wild herbs and broccoli. Since packet soups were no longer allowed in my shopping bag, I tried new recipes with surprising results. However, I often found it difficult to integrate the theory I gathered from books into my kitchen practice, many things I made out of habit had to change now, which was quite inconvenient, and it was a daily learning process – usually for the whole family. Familiar things have the bonus that, practised a thousand times, they become simple. I was lacking the instructions, advice, a cookery course with practical cooking tips.
Another problem for me back then was getting my hands on good bread. There was no organic baker here. So I tried to bake my own. Baking with yeast and baking powder worked well, but it there was always the issue of time for me. How do I integrate baking bread into my working day? I had to make compromises here, because I still lacked experience and routine. This is why I often used bread from the supermarket, which was sold as wholemeal bread. Unfortunately, it is only now that I know that this description does not have to have anything to do with

freshly ground whole grain, so the information is often incorrect. I had to learn that first, too. As well as bread and bread rolls, this problem also applies to cakes, pastries and pasta. If they are not made from wholemeal flours, they do not contain the important vital substances in their natural compound. They are then low in vital substances and are not suitable for my diet. I like to eat bread with herb butter or vegetable spreads. I also love bread or a "butter sandwich", as we Berliners call it, with a salad or soup.

A health day in Berlin

Together with friends we went to Berlin to a health event run by the Bruker house. I was very surprised at the number of people here who were familiar with this form of nutrition and who also lived this way. The interesting lectures reinforced the fact that my chosen path was right. I was particularly convinced that the Gesellschaft für Gesundheitsberatung GGB e.V. worked independently. I didn't see any advertising for medications or dietary supplements, and there were no free promotional gifts around either. I didn't feel cornered and didn't have to worry that this idea would burst like a bubble, because it was all about selling certain products. There was also no coffee, which I knew from my DCCV patient days. But there was a very tasty wholefood buffet! It had become clear to me after this event that I was only at the beginning and that there was still an awful lot for me to learn. For this reason I also took some information along with me, among other things, to a health week in Lahnstein.

My health continued to further improve in May and June. So I was able to reduce the Salofalk again without any problems. I was now only taking 1x Imurek and 3x Salofalk.

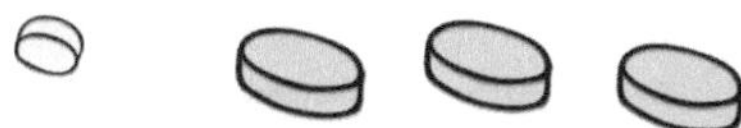

Adjustment problems

I had read something about gluten intolerance. Could my re-current flatulence, constipation and diarrhoea be related to this? Some days I had a firm, bloated belly, and I didn't know why. I would often eat too quickly and then wouldn't chew thoroughly enough and naturally the intestines need time to convert the superfine flour to real wholemeal. I therefore wanted to avoid gluten-containing cereals for a while and pre-dominantly use millet, buckwheat, amaranth, rice, corn and some oats for my fresh grain dish. I continued to eat wholemeal bread made of rye and spelt, but avoided eating very freshly baked bread. White and grey flour and all starchy foods, such as wheat noodles or wheat biscuits, were not on my menu, so it was not a completely gluten-free diet, but I saw it more as an adjustment aid for my body. I think it makes sense to take a few steps back where there is some form of disruption. I now also forego all dairy products, except butter, cream and eggs.

It is easy to bake with cereals containing less gluten. You can use buckwheat, amaranth, millet or maize instead of wheat or spelt for short pastry or for baking pancakes. Wholemeal bread rolls or breads are also successful if part of the wholemeal flour is replaced by gluten-free alternatives. However, the proportion of gluten-containing flour must predominate in order for the baked goods to be a success.

My problems decreased noticeably in the following weeks. I was surprised by my successes. It helped my very sensitive intestine to get used to the grain better. When I was feeling good and stable, I slowly increased the proportion of spelt for my fresh grain meal. From that point forward, I didn't notice my belly becoming distended. From this I've learned not to give up im-mediately, because it is important to observe the body well and to give it enough time.

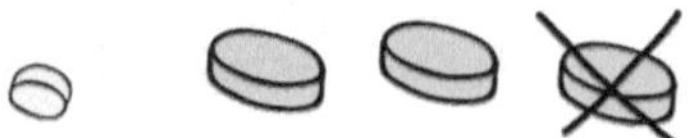

Other compatibilities

I now know that it isn't the individual food, but the composition of the food that causes many problems. Some food may be quickly demonised, but the cause of the problems lies in the combination with other foods, such as juices. Fruit, vegetable juices and cooked fruit do not belong in category of whole foods. The isolated sugar interferes with the nutrition of natural products. From my current experience, I know that many people have given up whole foods because they thought that juices were harmless and healthy, and bread or raw foods were blamed for flatulence. But it is the concentrated sugar and the lack of vital substances in the juices that cause intolerances.
Muesli bars, which also contain dried fruits, are also completely unsuitable for my sensitive intestines. Isolated and processed food must be strictly avoided.
I also needed some time to learn that heated fats could make whole foods intolerable. Frying fats, margarine and oils, which are produced under heat, are problematic. Heated fats no longer have their natural composition of fatty acids and can therefore considerably disturb the metabolism.
I guess intuitively, I didn't fry eggs, meat or fish at all, and even stir-fry vegetables were only steamed with water in the beginning. I used just a little olive oil only for baked vegetables, such as potatoes, beetroot, pumpkin or courgettes. However, fat is also an important flavour enhancer. Unheated fat in the form of butter, cold-pressed virgin oil or cream is only added once the dish has cooled down a little. In this way, the fat-soluble vitamins are preserved.
I read in Dr. Bruker's book: It's not that bad to have symptoms, it's bad when you don't know where they come from.

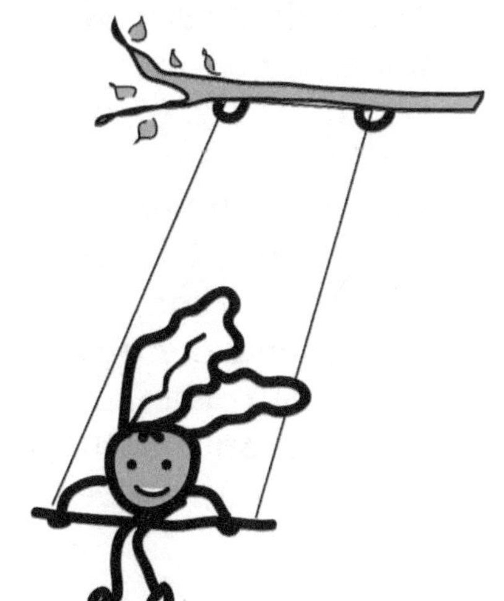

My health week

I couldn't shake the idea of the Health Week from my mind. The possibility of getting more information this way seemed to make sense to me, because it makes a difference whether one reads books or gets the knowledge at a seminar. I was also looking forward to having personal contact with like-minded people who are dealing with similar issues to me. This health week seemed be a suitable opportunity for this. I talked to Helmut about it, and he immediately supported me. In July there was still a place available and I registered straight away. I was enthusiastic about the range of events: whole foods were available throughout the week, and in the training kitchen you could take part in cooking and baking courses and get to know "1000 legal cooking tips". Kneipp hydrotherapy, the use of a hay flower sack, yoga, a public health consultation, sports, a demonstration of cupping therapy and a lecture entitled "All's fair in skin and hair" were part of the programme. As well as a lecture by Dr. Mathias Jung entitled
"My character – my fate". I was sure that I would get further with the many questions that concerned me.
I also wanted to learn more about baking bread with sourdough. And of course I hoped for medical advice because of my restless intestine, which continued to heal well, but was still very unstable. I get constipation more often, then diarrhoea again.

As the date approached, I got a little scared. It was my first trip since I'd been feeling better. But how stable will I be on such an exciting day? A friend had actually wanted to come along with me, but had to cancel at short notice. Will I be able manage this journey alone?
The journey to the station and the long train ride were still a problem for me at that time. I was still having about 3-5 bowel movements per day, usually in the morning. Stress and pressure, however, continued to play a specific role. What do I do if I'm standing on the platform with a suitcase and I have to go just as the train arrives? And on the long journey? Will it go

smoothly? I can't just leave my suitcase on the platform and rush off! As good as I am now in my daily life – I am usually at home. This trip was therefore a huge challenge!
In the morning I skipped breakfast, was able to leave the house on time and drove in the Regio to the train station in Berlin. The train to Koblenz was already at the platform waiting for me. From Koblenz I continued by bus to Lahnstein. I didn't get into difficulty once! Also during the week in Lahnstein I was doing so well that I was able to participate in the events without any problems. The only restriction I had was my morning difficulties with getting going, at seven o'clock in the training kitchen or the morning exercise? That hasn't quite worked out yet. Once I have reached my balance, there will be no more problems!
The attendees came from all over the country, as well as from Austria and Switzerland. I immediately felt at ease. Everyone who was there wanted to learn a lot, the atmosphere was relaxed and open-minded.
I particularly recall the introduction to Kneipp's treatments. This included a theory session discussing examples of application and a practical session, in which everyone could experience alternating blasts with a hose in a professional manner. They enables you to stimulate and strengthen your immune system.
Which pollutants cosmetics contain and how they affect the body was discussed in another lecture" Skin, hair and nails". Since I had already been experiencing problems with cosmetics and household chemical products, I was already aware of many of the issues. I will continue to deal with this in order to rule out sources of problems for the future. A practical experience is the hay flower bag. It is heated by steam and placed directly on the body, so that the hay flowers can unfold their full effect of relaxation.
 The lectures with Mathias Jung "Hans, my hedgehog" and the "Frog King – A hot relationship" were particularly entertaining.
I also managed to get a doctor's appointment with Dr. Birmanns. He spent a whole hour listening to me and I told him about my illness, the unauthorised reduction in medication and

my current state of health. He was not surprised by this success and didn't make me feel irresponsible at having arbitrarily reduced my medication. His only comment was that it was my body, and that it was normal that I should take care of it myself. I used this opportunity to talk to a holistic doctor about my current symptoms, especially the fragile nature of my intestines when using the phone or under deadline pressure. I also discussed difficulties getting going in the mornings.

I knew that my intestines had changed due to the flare-ups, much cannot be repaired. It often feels to me like it's swollen, which makes it act like a blockage. I was very hopeful that these problems could be solved.

Dr. Birmanns asked many questions and gave me just as many answers. He prescribed homoeopathic remedies for my irritable bowel, which reacts to stress with "I won't let you go anywhere". Aloe D12 (2-3 x five drops) and Phosphorus C30 once a week five globules in the morning on an empty stomach, for three days, if a reaction occurs after the first administration, read the instructions.

I was glad that I chose to come on this week and had overcome it; I had come a long way. This experience also gave me another piece of security. I came home with many new impressions and I knew that I was on the right track.

One topic that was particularly important to me now was to organise my life. Mathias Jung's lectures had reinforced the fact that only I can make a difference myself. I need a healthier work and leisure routine, as well as a routine that includes activity and rest. And I will learn to take more care of myself. I want to protect and love the little girl inside me. It also made me also realise how lucky I am with my family and that my love and family are the most important things to me.

Using freshly ground grain continued to keep me busy. The fresh grain can be used in many ways in the kitchen, especially in baking, of course. Once back home, I made sourdough with great enthusiasm to make bread. I had enjoyed the bread in Lahnstein – could I make that too? However, using sourdough, which I now wanted to try out, turned out to be much more difficult. I just didn't develop the right feeling for the dough, especially since I had only limited time at my disposal. After several attempts I gave up. I guess I couldn't give the dough the attention it needed. The dough dried up, overflowed or started to grow mould because I often forgot to take care of it. I found it difficult to maintain the right temperature for the bacteria over the full period of several days. So I planned to attend a bread baking course at a later date.

But everyone was very happy with the breads and cakes that I made from yeast dough, and I enjoyed making these treats.

The problem with refined sugar

Why is sugar such a problem? I've learned a lot about that here: the refining process isolates pure cane sugar from the natural sugar beet in a multi-stage chemical process (beet sugar is also known as cane sugar). During the process, vital substances are completely lost. The excessive consumption of refined sugar leads to deficiency symptoms and intolerances, since the body needs vitamin B and calcium to process sugar. This causes permanent damage to our body over time. Since most diseases take 20 to 30 years to develop, the connection with nutrition is difficult to see.

A particular difficulty nowadays is that sugar is present in large quantities in processed foods. And not just in sweet foods, but also in packet soups, spiced gherkins, meat salads or tinned fish. For me it was a long learning process for me to understand how to avoid these things completely and that my food and cakes could still taste good.

Only when I use raw and fresh products exclusively, can I avoid this "hidden" sugar found in processed foods. I also got rid of the habit of "sweetening", the sweet addition when cooking and baking. The amount got smaller. I knew that when I used sugar, it was never good for me! To my amazement, however, eliminating sugar was never a problem in terms of taste, the real problem was the persistent habits. I first had to develop the confidence that a recipe without sugar was okay, and that my sense of taste would have to return to what it once was, which was a remarkable experience for me. I have rediscovered the variety of flavours offered by natural products and have found that the taste of fresh vegetables cannot be replaced by industrially processed products and artificial flavourings. The standard taste created by sugar, salt and flavour enhancers was really no loss at all! If I needed anything sweetening, then I would use honey or ripe fruits. In recipes, I replaced sugar with honey by halving the amount. Ripe fruits or nut flour further reduced the honey. The family also found it easy to make a friend of honey in place of sugar.

Sugar should never be replaced by sweeteners or fructose. Sorbitol is particularly harmful as a sugar substitute in many low-calorie foods (e.g. sugar-free chewing gums). It is broken down into short chain fatty acids and gases (hydrogen, methane, carbon dioxide) in the large intestine and often causes diarrhoea and unpleasant gas formation.

I don't need to eat sweet treats now. I now know that my sugar consumption is a significant part of my illness. I was always slim and for this very reason I probably thought I didn't have to hold back. I used to love sweet treats and would eat them as "anxiety food", "comfort food", as an "energizer", or simply because they looked so good and the fruity flavours would shout out to me, "Have more"!

Holiday in Hungary

A holiday again at last. After our house-building project, we put off any holidays for a year. In August we planned a holiday in Hungary. We were looking for a rural holiday with riding facilities. We found a romantic holiday resort: a modern country estate with a pool and a pretty apartment for us. Josefine is an avid horse rider and rides regularly. Besides an indoor riding arena, there were also plenty of opportunities for cross-country rides. We also found the place ideal for Snoopy.

As a child I had spent several summer holidays in this beautiful country, so I was sure that the food would not be a problem for me. I remembered fresh tomatoes, peppers, corn, peaches, apricots and much more, so I really didn't have any concerns. And so we booked full-board accommodation.

But it all turned out to be very different. In the meantime, the world had been turned upside down here in Hungary too. The eating culture of this beautiful holiday and equestrian farm was not at all so rural. There was only tinned fruit, there were no fresh vegetables, the mashed potatoes tasted like dry powder, and everything was prepared with lots of sugar. There were certainly no wholemeal products. I was shocked. Instead of sticking to good Hungarian, fresh food, the chef experimented with the new western ready-made and industrial foods products. This "price" was too high for me, I opted out of the meals. I didn't want to risk jeopardising my hard-earned health. My family stayed, especially since we only had a small kitchen in our apartment.

So I headed off to visit the local farmers' market with great anticipation. But even what I found there was not what I had hoped for! There was a marketplace with empty stalls. An elderly lady was selling some onions, and a second was selling a bowl of walnuts. Where were the cheerful, black-haired Magyars from my childhood with peppers, cucumbers, tomatoes and boiled corn? My dream of fresh fruit and vegetables and a spicy fish soup was over, I had to admit that realistically. But there was a shop in the neighbouring village, what other choice did I have than to shop there? I simply made the best of it; I got what I needed here, plenty of fruit, vegetables, cream, sour cream and white bread – there was no other bread. But everything did me good. There was no deterioration in my condition during the holiday. I kept my medication unchanged over that period.

To be on the safe side, I went to the local pharmacy and handed in another prescription for some Salofalk, which was even in stock! Instead of EUR 412, here it cost 9534.00 Forint, the equivalent of EUR 79.18.

Our dog, Snoopy, fell in love for the first time in Hungary. A German shepherd bitch had turned his head. Day and night he stood at our bay window, his paws on the radiator, looking out of the window and howling at his highest pitch. The Hungarian language wasn't difficult for him, and love moves mountains.

Since I had fallen off my horse while riding in the arena (I wanted to go straight ahead, the horse had decided to turn), it gave us a good excuse to go to the thermal mud baths in Héviz. The warm healing mud is particularly recommended for rheumatism and aching limbs, and we used the day extensively to pamper ourselves.

This holiday was good for me and the whole family. And I gained the confidence that even in unforeseeable situations it is possible to find a sensible nutritional solution for me. There is no need for complicated ingredients to eat naturally.

Back home Helmut had a surprise for me. He had bought me an electric grain mill. It was made of solid beech wood and equipped with a corundum millstone. This mill took place of honour in our kitchen and from then on became my most important kitchen appliance.

Children and wholefood cuisine

Of course, nutrition and the health of my family are very important to me. I'm often asked whether all family members now have to eat my "special diet", even the children, or whether I make two dinners. I never asked myself that question. This was probably because I was thrilled from the beginning at how much we all enjoy whole foods and how good they make us feel!

Everybody likes the fresh grain dish. My fresh raw vegetable salads and vegetable platters are also popular – I often feel that the colourful vegetables are responsible for my good mood. I have always managed to convince even stubborn refusers of raw food with a good dressing.

I was also very successful with both children with my soups, ir-

relevant of whether it was a cream soup or a vegetable stew. They were a warm complement after a large salad platter. With some croutons or toasted wholemeal bread and fresh herbs, they were very popular with the children and still are today with the grandchildren.
Nobody can resist wholemeal bread and freshly baked rolls. There is something very special about the smell of good bread permeating the house, it gives you such a warm, homely feeling.

To start with, it was difficult with the darker cake mixtures and pizza doughs. The kids didn't find it quite so cool. However, the transition can be made slowly by just replacing one part flour with wholemeal flour. This allows the eye and palate to adjust and get used to it. Of course I only ate one piece of cake and an apple.
The family's enthusiasm for baguettes, white rolls and toast remained nevertheless, though it had decreased considerably. I was pleased at how tasty everyone found my wholemeal rolls but I did understand my children's desire to eat "white" rolls. Incidentally, these days, light rolls are once again one of my "favourites", I bake them from nutritious Kamut or a mixture of spelt and Kamut.

The children have different tastes and preferences, but we always managed to find a compromise. Nobody had to eat anything they didn't like, there were no obligations and certainly no rules. I saw it as an opportunity for my new cooking habits to select and prepare the food so that it excited everyone.
And children always learn from their parents. Since Helmut is open-minded to new things, the children didn't link the change in nutrition to my illness, but instead took it as a positive experience and reacted to it in a casual manner. Maybe that's the secret. The times we share in the kitchen are the highlight of the day, because we are simply together. We talk, chop and grate – and it smells so good. The change in menu between traditional dishes and "my creations" creates confidence. This means that children, given the necessary encouragement, from

an early age, are able to handle knives and pans themselves and to put their ideas into practice in the kitchen. And they do, and they inspire me too.

In my experience, the simpler the dishes, the better. Many so-called "peasant meals" are a treat, lovingly prepared with fresh, seasonal ingredients.
Crucial to the preparation are the fresh ingredients and a little imagination. That is why I changed traditional, popular family recipes, such as roast potatoes, potatoes, linseed oil and quark and lentils to vegetable fillings, vegetable casseroles with rice, grains or pasta, fricassee with rice, egg with spinach or with asparagus. I then used potatoes in skins instead of peeled potatoes and wholemeal rice instead of husked rice, and of course wholemeal grain instead of superfine flour. Omelettes or vegetable pizzas are also easy to make with wholemeal flour. One of the initial hurdles was wholemeal pasta. We didn't like many varieties, they were just too mushy. I always like pasta to be firm to the bite! These days, however, there are so many better varieties made from wholemeal durum wheat or spelt, which we love to eat because we find they taste so good.
I now find white pasta tasteless – my sense of taste has changed. Much of what I didn't like as a child has now become a delicacy in adulthood. Capers, cabbage rolls, onion cakes, olives, raisins, those were the absolute no-go's for me back then! So I know just how our tastes can change throughout life. I try to give every dish that doesn't get the full approval of the family a second and third chance by swapping ingredients around and preparing it differently.

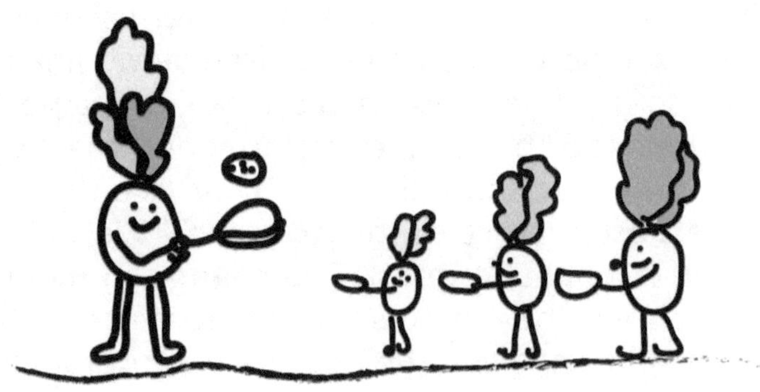

Our children are involved in buying and preparing our food. They can choose the vegetables we use, and their likes and dislikes are taken into account. Pizza dough or small vegetable pies that they can make themselves always go down well. A successful wholemeal yeast dough is never safe from hungry little mouth in our kitchen. They like to make their own omelettes or pancakes filled with vegetables and served with spicy sauce or garlic cream.

Colourful pancakes (omelettes) baked with wild garlic, carrots or beetroot are also very popular with our grandchildren and encourage them to experiment. And our potato cakes taste completely different when I make them from grated carrots, parsnips or pumpkin. Soups can be made more colourful by adding beetroot, pumpkin and red cabbage. Regional vegetables can lead to completely new combinations and taste experiences, such as a winter borscht of cabbage and turnips.

When I think about it now, this is a positive side to my illness and I am grateful for it. As a result, our children have also become very consciously aware of alternatives to general nutrition, which is considered to be healthy. They have experienced that fresh tastes better and that enjoyment sometimes requires a little more effort and love.

Three of our children (now 37, 35 and 29 years old) still don't drink coffee. None of them has ever smoked. They have always been interested in sports, so coffee and smoking did not fit with their life plan. These are, I think, good prerequisites to developing their interest in this form of nutrition. The fact that my family has gone along with me has been an enormous help. It has made me happy and is pivotal in why I am getting better and better.

What about meat and fish?

I don't want to demonise the enjoyment of meat and fish, since both have been part of our diet from the outset. But there is the issue of the amount that is consumed. Looking back at the eating habits of our ancestors, the Sunday roast was still something special.

However, the significantly increased consumption of meat has many effects on our lives. The unlimited daily availability of meat at the lowest prices inevitably leads to cruel mass livestock farming. The animals have to grow quickly, and the cost of housing and food mustn't be too high – the result is stressed meat with a high water content that does not taste good. Often this deficit is covered in the trade by pre-seasoned products.

An even more critical aspect to be evaluated is the use of more and more antibiotics in the large fattening farms. Today, 40 times more antibiotics are used in intensive livestock farming than in German hospitals. We consume some of it when we eat the meat, the rest is excreted in the manure into the groundwater and comes from there into our food chain. This unwanted and uncontrolled long-term medication inevitably leads to allergies. The intensive use of antibiotics is also common in the breeding of fish in so-called aquacultures. And there is another factor that speaks out against excessive meat production and mass livestock farming: 40 percent of the world's grain and soya crops are processed into animal feed. If this amount were given directly into the food cycle of humans, it would solve many problems of worldwide hunger. Germany is also one of the importers of grain and soya for animal feed production.

There is another important health issue. In many diseases, it is essential to restrict the consumption of animal protein, e.g. in motor system disorders, in diabetes and in so-called allergic diseases. In many cases, healing or at least an improvement can be achieved in the initial stage. This is particularly true for primary chronic polyarthritis and other forms of chronic rheumatoid arthritis. A very strict adherence to an animal protein-free diet is necessary for neurodermatitis – an otherwise incurable disease. But animal protein should also be avoided or severely restricted in cases of skin diseases, recurrent infections, cardiovascular diseases and diabetes. The increase in these diseases over the last 100 years is also due to the growing consumption of animal products.

We have agreed in the family to eat less and less fish or meat, and this works well. Cooking with whole foods provides new positive taste experiences every day; we really don't miss meat.

The need for meat is often justified by talk of a possible protein deficiency. How important is protein for our health? And how do I meet my protein requirements if I eat mostly raw food? Apart from animal products such as milk, yoghurt, quark, cheese, eggs, sausage, fish and meat, high-quality protein is found in sufficient quantities in vegetables and is particularly abundant in legumes.

Another problem is that we usually consume heated protein. Which means it is no longer natural, but denatured. I learnt this in my later courses. And since raw meat and fish are not an alternative and most milk products are only available once they have been treated at high or ultra-high temperatures. So I decided to largely forego these too.
It is important to me to enjoy the majority of my vegetables raw, because this is the only way to get enough VIRGIN protein. Luckily, the raw food does me good. I don't think my body is lacking anything. I don't want to destroy this new balance, and I'm very careful.
I use yoghurt and quark occasionally, but only if it has a high fat content. As we know, fat does not make you fat, and I tell myself that where there is fat, there can't be any protein. I tolerate butter and cream well. Butter contains only 0.5 percent protein in 98 per cent fat, and cream contains only 2.5 per cent protein, which is rarely a problem. Since I mainly eat raw food, I don't have to worry about eating excess fat by adding butter and cream. Plus, I like them, especially when they are fresh and well chilled!

Good prospects

In September, my doctor performed a sonography (ultrasound), which revealed: unremarkable findings.
The colonoscopy showed: moderate haemorrhoids tinged with

blood, normal coloured mucous membrane intact throughout the entire colon, with no pathological findings. Post inflammatory changes in the descending colon, florid ulceration in the first 25 cm – bleeding only on contact with the endoscope. Grade II haemorrhoids as an additional source of bleeding. The recommendation was: continue 3 x 2 Claversal (as before) and continue 3 x Imurek, to maintain remission, for a further 14 days continue Betnesol enemas, and review as necessary. Additionally ferro sanol duodenal (225 mg iron(II)glycine-sulphate complex).

My doctor didn't know that I was only taking 1x Imurek and 2x Salofalk daily. I avoided the discussion, since I haven't felt this well and alive in the last six years. I knew that if I could identify further stable improvements in my condition, I would be able to reduce the medication even further.
Apart from everyday conditions, the following symptoms have disappeared completely since changing my diet: dry skin and dry mucous membranes, eczema, hair loss, water retention, various allergic reactions and pain in the hip joints, rheumatism in the hands and dry eyes. In addition, my skin has changed for the better, it is now very calm, fine-pored and soft. I no longer have dry, itchy or greasy areas. My hair is much thicker again, the grey hair has completely disappeared. While I was taking the medication, there were times when the right side of my hair and the back of my head were completely grey.
How can I not feel at ease with these successes?
I told my doctor that I still had enough Betnesol, which was true, and that I only wanted to use it when necessary. He agreed. I always make sure that I have enough medication for emergencies or that I have a valid prescription in reserve, if necessary.

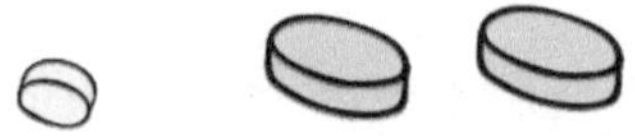

At the beginning of October, after another three months, I sealed the last pack of Imurek. It was a great feeling. I had no concerns. It was just nice to completely entrust my body to my own immune system again. It's going to be all right now. I didn't notice any health issues over the weeks since stopping this medication either. I now only take 2x1 tablet Salofalk. This is now available as granules, which is more pleasant to take and disperses better in the intestine.

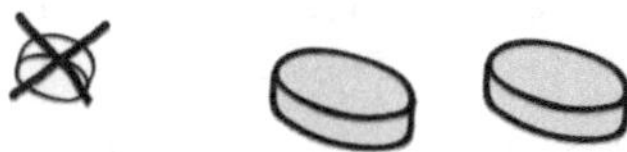

I still have problems with flatulence or a bloated stomach. In October, my doctor diagnosed chronic diarrhoea. At the moment, however, I am most burdened with the symptoms of haemorrhoids, which refuse to settle down.

Cabbage and onions?

In previous diets, onions, cabbage and pulses were well-known for being on the no-go list. After I switched to whole foods, I cut down my intake of these. I only started my diet using the vegetables that I knew I could digest, so kohlrabi and carrots. I slowly expanded my repertoire. Cabbage, peas, lentils, onions and beans were at the back of this
"queue". After a year, once I had integrated almost all the different vegetables and fruits as part of my cooking habits and once I knew I could tolerate them well, I started to experiment. Sauerkraut, red cabbage, cauliflower, broccoli and Brussels sprouts were added to raw vegetable salads or soups. Cabbage and onions were also ideal for casseroles, vegetable pies and vegetable stir-fries. Savoy cabbage or white cabbage tasted good braised, raw or in colourful vegetable stir-fries. I also included onion tart, onion soups, grilled, stuffed or stewed onions in my menu. And I didn't notice any serious problems. I had the

same outcome with pulses. Lentils and mung beans taste great sprouted in a salad, or I sprinkle them over a ready-to-serve vegetable dish, lentil salad and also chilli con carne: I also tolerated these dishes well.

I used chickpea flour to experiment with baking flatbreads and bread. It can also be used to make smooth spreads. I didn't notice any health problems. These foods naturally cause a little more flatulence. As the saying goes: "Every little bean makes a sound". This is not an illness. It's just a good sign that our intestinal bacteria are working hard. These are happy farts. Just listen to the difference!

Cabbage, onions and pulses are foods rich in vital substances and proteins. I find these very tasty and they enrich our meals, especially in winter. Sauerkraut and pickled vegetables make a wonderful daily addition to good winter cooking! Animal protein can therefore be replaced sufficiently and nutritiously.

It's the beginning of November. A year ago I started to change my diet to a nutritious wholefood diet. I've been getting better every week since then. In all those previous years, I have never felt as good as I do this year. Back then, healthy phases lasted a few months at best. Even then, they were achieved through taking high-doses of drugs.

Now I feel well enough to do things on my own again. I laugh and sing and can move freely for an unlimited period of time. I enjoy my family and I'm able to make it through my extensive working day.

I cut out another tablet of Salofalk. I'm still taking the very last tablet up until 31st December, I decided.

Do you have to suffer to be beautiful?

At the beginning of December I had some minor problems with my face. Again the eczema was treated with Remederm Widmer Rp. Leuckichthyol/Dermatop ointment.

I was being careful. Where had this come from? What was my

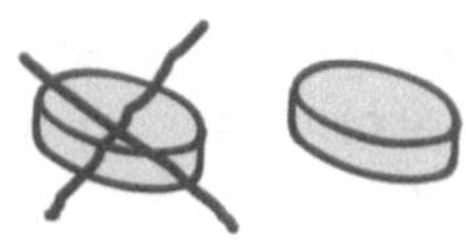

body telling me? I had already noticed on several occasions that the use of cosmetics causes conjunctivitis and skin irritation, especially on my face. So now I wanted to find out the exact cause.

I not only had to worry about my diet, but also about how to deal with cosmetics, I knew that. How much do I need and what is really necessary, good and useful for me, and what can and must I do without? In the following weeks I carried out some "self-experiments".

For a year we have been dancing regularly. It was on these occasions especially, I tested the reactions caused by the various pots, tubes and vials that I had. After a short time I started to feel the skin on my face become tight, itchy and red and my eyes started to inflame. Once I stopped using all the creams and cosmetics, the problems were less severe on the days that followed. This was no longer an acceptable solution for me, I wanted to find the cause.

First, I tested my nail polish. I wore just this and no other cosmetics. After just two hours I felt my skin start to tighten. A light prickling and tingling. My eyelids became drier, a pink area appeared on my neck. The next morning my face was blotchy and red. I removed every last bit of the nail polish. The symptoms decreased again by the evening and disappeared completely after three days.

After two weeks, I tried it again with the same results. A third but shorter attempt also confirmed my suspicion. I knew now that I shouldn't use nail polish anymore. I didn't test whether these symptoms were caused by specific brands; I assumed formaldehyde played a role here, but I didn't want to do any further tests, especially as I couldn't see very well because of the conjunctivitis that it cause and it affected my ability to work each time. I was aware that my intestinal mucosa, in other words my immune system, is currently being rebuilt. I assume this also applies to all other mucous membranes and connective membranes in my body. So I'm going to avoid any further exposure!

Fragrances were my next subject to address. I've never been a fan of spraying fragrance daily because I had previously had skin reactions and I didn't like the alien smell on my body. It didn't feel like me and I just wanted to smell like myself again. I found it unpleasant when someone used a lot of perfume and the inevitable smell it left in my office, apartment or on my clothes. I would then become fuzzy-headed and I felt like my space wasn't my own anymore. I am obviously not only very sensitive, but also a very odour-sensitive person. When I used perfume or perfumed creams, my skin reacted, even if I only wet my clothes or hair. This would trigger the familiar symptoms. Previously, it had never been a reason for me to stop using them, because I assumed my body would handle them.

I also had problems with deodorants. Heavily weeping, red spots would form under my armpits and would last for several weeks. I would also get skin tags. These symptoms also disappeared completely.

Make-up, especially near my eyes, and powders cause me problems immediately after application. The consequence was that my general health suffered because I could only see to a limited extent. Closing my eyes didn't bring any relief, the problems usually only disappeared the next day. So, I looked for alternatives in the organic food store that were more compatible.

By reducing my health-burdening substances, I hoped to be able to avoid many problems in the future, because obviously my immune system was becoming weakened by them. I often felt like I was sometimes trusting advertising and media hype more than my own body – I wanted to change that.

On 28 December I had an appointment with my gynaecologist who diagnosed the disease six years ago. She was truly amazed at how well the colitis was now healing. She found my change of diet very interesting and said, if it helped me, I should definitely continue with it. This was the first time that a "conventional doctor" encouraged me and acknowledged the role of my diet. I got the feeling that she believed me! She saw that I was doing well and felt that had I had gained radiance through this experience. She told me that too and it made me feel good. The findings were: Improvement of ulcerative colitis through diet."

Medication costs in 2002: 1300,57 Euro

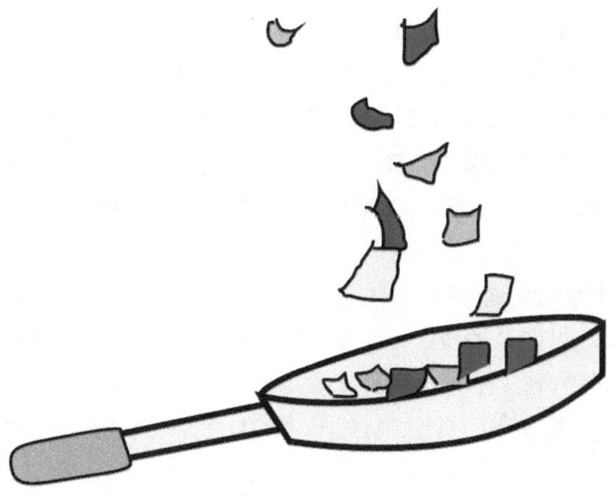

2003

Listening to my body

At the beginning of February we spent a few days on the wintry Baltic Sea. In stormy wind and blue sky we hiked over the island of Rügen. I really pampered my immune system. After the long and stormy hikes, we made extensive use of the sauna in our holiday home. I enjoyed being able to experience a holiday so freely and carefree!

Then things took a very different turn. A phone call from our office turned the world upside down. We had to make a decision immediately and stopped our holiday at once. In the life of the self-employed it is quite normal for there to be ups and downs, both small and large. What is particularly difficult is that you are always personally affected by it, without any filter.

Four days later, the bleeding and the pain started. I still had enough Salofalk anti-inflammatories and prescribed myself 3x1 tablet daily. When the pain increased despite this and I wasn't feeling any better after three days, I took a low dose of Decortin for 5 days, which I also still had. I wanted to stop the bleeding in its tracks. I was having up to ten bowel movements a day. I changed my diet back to PURE raw vegetables. It took five more days, then the bleeding started to subside. After almost four weeks, the symptoms had completely disappeared.

That was a warning sign for me. It really scared me. And it was clear that not only permanent stress, but also sudden stress weakens my immune system so much that my intestines suffer from it. My intestinal brain was responding to overload. In the future I will have to learn to deal with setbacks in such a way that they put less strain on my body. This is perhaps the most difficult task that still lies ahead of me.

In March I wanted to tackle the unpleasant issue of haemorrhoids, which are accompanied by constipation and then bleeding. I assumed these to be a consequence of a change in the
tissue due to the long-standing illness. I was now feeling stable
enough to solve this last problem. My doctor referred me to a
specialist who was could ablate the haemorrhoids.
Since I no longer struggled to travel to Berlin to see the doctor,
I wasted no time in going. By April, after three treatments, they
had healed to a large extent. Another change for the better.

It's May, and I'm doing well. I don't take medication anymore
and I weigh 57 kg again. I eat a fresh grain dish every day for
breakfast and a large vegetable and fruit snack in the office at
noon, plus wholemeal bread.
I don't consume any industrially processed foods that may contain unknown substances. I "cleaned up" my kitchen cabinets
and disposed of everything containing sugar, salt and artificial
additives. These included toppings and soups in packets, ready-
made flour mixtures of all kinds, most tinned and frozen ready
meals, some spice mixtures and spice sauces. This has created
the space that I now need for the variety of grain, seeds and
pulses.

As our cooking habits continue to change, I can now eat with
my family more often. But the good old habits are always lurk-
ing. The initial extra effort is to be expected if you are to gain
sufficient new experiences! The fact that Helmut likes to cook
makes it a lot easier for me. His cheerful disposition helps to
overcome many initial problems. He went over my new recipe
ideas and then told me straight away what he didn't like, what
he didn't want to eat or if he liked something else. That was a
big help to me. Cooking became a new hobby for us, it is a challenge to create things that always have the promise of a new
pleasure. A hobby that holds many discoveries for the family as
a whole, because it also infects the children when they see how
we "negotiate". It also meant that our dog, Snoopy, could be
with us, lying right in the middle, so that it was impossible to
get past him. Though that provided good entertainment, be-

cause even the big children sat close on the kitchen floor and played together.
Learning about wholefood cuisine isn't that difficult once you understand the principle of naturalness. It is much more difficult to part with old eating and cooking habits. A great help here is having the opportunity to learn about wholefood cooking through courses. I didn't know about these opportunities back then; today I'm more than happy to learn from them.

I feel like this is the best time of my life. I feel powerful, beautiful and healthy. I'm happy, I'm working a lot and I love it. I try to spend my free time with the family, and doing my hobbies: painting, dancing and gardening.
This year, for the first time, I organised a large exhibition with my art group, which was a great success.

The follow-up examination on 1st October with my gastroenterologist showed: "...no anal bleeding in known colitis".
I no longer have skin problems or allergies and joint pain is very rare. However, there are days when I have pain in my wrists. I think this is due to using a mouse on the computer. This is the reason why I'm planning to further reduce the proportion of animal protein in my diet in the future.

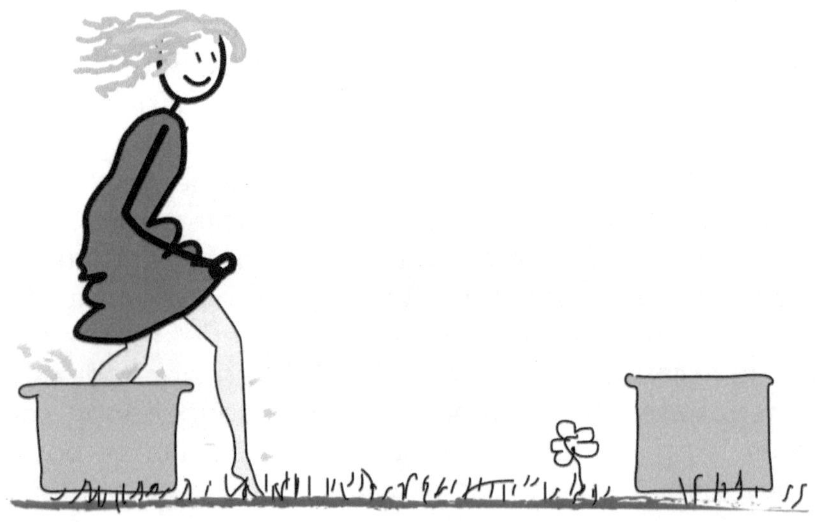

In addition to eating whole foods, taking lots of exercise and relaxation, toughening up has also become an important pillar of my health.

I paced barefoot and vigorously across the lawn in my garden every day, even in winter. It's what I called my early morning walk. Here I can draw on my knowledge from Health Week. Alternating warm-cold arm baths or jets of water to the arm promote blood circulation and stimulate self-healing powers. I also use gymnastics and stretching of the ligaments as therapy against these problems.

Medication costs in 2003: 0 Euro.

2004

Slower successes

This spring we had great business success! After working for several weeks on an extensive presentation, we won a very interesting client. It involved rural life in Brandenburg and producers of regional products. I was particularly happy about this assignment, since this topic has close links to my new eating, shopping and living habits. The project involves designing and producing flyers, catalogues and posters to inform people about the region and its agricultural products. In addition, harvest festivals, for example, needed help to advertise themselves. We needed a lot of good photos for these orders, so we were now on the road a lot in the countryside. I was able to combine my hobbies of photography and cycling with the discovery and buying of regional products. A combination I like very much. Even though these new activities mainly took place at the weekends, the exercise meant that my work was varied and balanced. Cycling is becoming more and more important for me; I feel very comfortable doing it.

One subject that I can't get leave alone is bringing more calmness into my everyday office life. I have been able to delegate some tasks to employees. I try to plan and organise my workdays more carefully, but all too often that doesn't comply with clients' expectations: an immediate, quick solution to usually large-scale orders. Unforeseen technical problems or employees who are absent for several days ensure that my good intentions often just flutter away. So reorganisation is needed; I only find the time to catch up at night. Then, if I really want to relax, I have to fit in the extra work elsewhere. In these recurring situations I often feel worn out between the overpowering demands and then my battery empties. As a self-employed person, you are responsible for everything, and in my profession there are no standards, nothing is prefabricated. Everything I design for my clients goes through a development process, I come up with the ideas and the implementation and organisation of production follow. That's what I love about my job, and a certain compulsion for perfection is part of it. But how much perfection is really necessary? Quite a lot, because every mistake in this process I pay for myself, this fact is part of my almost 30 years of professional experience.

I maintain my eating habits, however there are always exceptions. But I feel very healthy and think that I can eat what is offered at events, for example.
There is a daily portion of fresh grain in the office. I soak the grain at home early on, and I freshly cut the fruit in the tea kitchen at the office. The time required for this lunch is manageable. But are we on a trip and don't have time for that, we have to eat something on the way. In the afternoon there is a big, colourful vegetable platter, and if I don't have time to eat that, a bag of carrots is waiting in the fridge, so that I am able to feel balanced and well throughout the long office day. I no longer experience those phases of severe fatigue after eating. I don't need sweet treats in the office anymore. This is a very impressive change for me. I suspect the cause in the sweet fresh grain dish, which supplies me with an even amount of sugar over a relatively long period of time. I remember well how I often was unable to continue working without chocolate because I felt so exhausted.
In summer it is often very warm in the office and there is ice cream for everyone. Although it didn't cause me any problems, I have to say that this kind of treat is nowadays a rare exception. I know it's not good for me, so I don't see it as a loss. But there are more alternatives to discover!

We have a warm meal in the evening, even though I come home very late, it is cooked daily. It may not be healthy, but it is our way of life, and I feel comfortable with it. Chopping of the evening salad and cooking help me to leave the working day behind me. I can switch off and relax, especially since the result of the cooking always includes a reward for having had a good day.

I love the feeling when I come home in the evening, walk through my garden with a basket and look for what I can prepare for the day. I collect what is ripe and looks good, and that's when the idea for the dish comes into being. It is my voyage of discovery that I happily enjoy.

For me, cooking has a lot to do with my love of nature. The way in which fresh, seasonal products are used is a challenge, and I notice that in traditional, simple recipes this idea is often perfectly implemented. Braised cucumbers with new potatoes, dill and fresh tomatoes? Sour cream with wild herbs, linseed oil and potatoes from the garden? Millet with tomatoes, cucumbers, peppers, garlic and fresh herbs? The ideas come almost by themselves... It gives me a good feeling to live in harmony with nature in this way, to coordinate my gardening and my eating habits and to get involved. If I can successfully combine these things, I develop a feeling of satisfaction, which in turn slows me down.

Medication costs in 2004: 0 Euro.

2005

Longing for Spring

I feel drained by the end of winter now. Maybe because it is more difficult to eat a diet rich in vital substances that it is in summer. The supply of fruit and vegetables in the supermarket is mainly determined by products from the South. Much of it looks very tempting, but is less fresh because of the long transportation routes, and I avoid it because it's probably also more contaminated with pesticides. For citrus fruits that do not come from organic farming, I notice immediately if the peel has been treated. Even hand washing them after peeling doesn't get rid of the pesticides. Apples and carrots, turnips and cabbage are therefore my most important raw food supplier in winter.
Nevertheless, I am symptom-free. I wait longingly for spring and the beginning of the gardening season, when the table is set with a greater variety again.
In order to grow our own vegetables, we decided to get a greenhouse. Six square metres is not much, but it allows you to harvest your own salad as early as the end of March. This is followed by kohlrabi, cauliflower, cucumbers, aubergines and peppers. Tomatoes are one of those things that prefer to be alone in the greenhouse. They like a dry climate but want their feet to get wet. But you can harvest them in the greenhouse until the end of October.

I'm feel good and am happy with my body and my appearance. I am happy and like to accept everything as it is. 44 is a beautiful age. I have enough strength again to do everything I intend to do, and there is no problem that I cannot solve. A friend who has known me for 35 years said to me, "Micha, you've completely changed, you now radiate so much self-confidence!"
We have also raised the pace in our dancing. The dance school

has been superseded by the dance sports club. We learn lots of new step combinations, and at the same time we pay much more attention to technique and posture. In a sense, mind and body are burdened more at the same time. The smaller groups also mean that the dance teacher is able to supervise more closely and can correct mistakes immediately. Sometimes it is quite annoying to have to repeat the same step ten or fifteen times. We are then rewarded when others on the "normal dance floor" gaze at us in admiration.

How can I find my working rhythm?

Permanent ongoing stress was certainly one of the causes that led to the outbreak of the disease in my case. As a self-employed person, that certainly cannot always be avoided, but it can be reduced by reorganising the work. Based on this insight, I tried in the following weeks and months to reorganise my work and life rhythm. That sounds simple, but it isn't. Finishing work at 8pm is on my wish list every day. In reality, of course, this rarely happens. A fundamental experience I've had is: I need sufficient breaks between the individual stages of my work in order to cope with strenuous tasks well and quickly. If this change is missing, my effectiveness decreases rapidly over the course of the day. Certainly not a new insight, but it was important for me to discover and experience it for myself. Only in being able to find your own work rhythm will you be able to avoid unnecessary stress.
While I'm an early bird, my husband is more of a night owl. This definitely helps him to combine his work in the office with his social commitments.
When his evening events are over, he drives back to the office and does what the pixies didn't want to do. Where does he get the energy for these additional tasks? If you want to change something, you have to get involved. Grumbling doesn't help. I would like to support him, but my battery is all too often flat in the evening. Do I work differently than he does? I've had an

easy childhood and never been exposed to such an extremely high degree of responsibility. It was very different for him. Through his difficult experiences, he has learned resilience and composure.

Another solution is to reduce the size of the company. This would reduce the number of orders required to pay employees at the end of the month. At the same time, I would have fewer projects to look at and would have more time for the design tasks that give me the greatest satisfaction. I think it's worth thinking about.
In recent years, nine young people have successfully completed their apprenticeships in our company. We have now decided to bring this to a close. During my illness, my work as an instructor, was very stressful because my intestines had determined my pace of life.
Regular progress meetings, work instructions and presentations of projects; these obligations took up a large part of my daily working time. I enjoyed it and thanks to the mostly exemplary work of the trainees I was able to ensure the high quality of the work. All trainees completed their training with good and very good results. Unfortunately, the completion of the training was for most only a springboard to study, which meant that we lost well trained employees again shortly after the end of the apprenticeship. I had a hard time dealing with that every time.
Now I want to transfer this time to other tasks – or should I just do nothing?

I discovered watercolour painting. The lightness of this technique and the wonderful luminosity of the colours appeal to me. With the help of water you can lighten the colours. When different colours meet, chance continues to paint, creating structures that look like water, sky or fields or ones that are simply beautiful. If I wait until the colours are dry, I can put a new translucent colour layer over them, thereby creating three-dimensionality and vividness. White paper should stand still, then it develops its own charm. I now succeed with ease in the looseness that painting requires.

Working with watercolours requires little preparation and can be done practically anywhere. At home I converted part of my room into a studio. The work I have begun remains on the table. The pictures can dry and I can look at them or continue working on them at any time. It's mostly moods or feelings that I put on paper. Painting is relaxing for me.

Medication costs in 2005: 0 Euro.

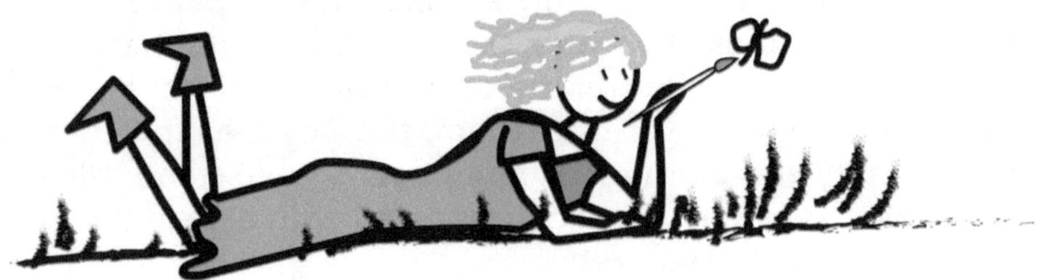

2006

A silly idea

Like every year after a long winter, I long for spring. I eat salad and vegetables regularly and try to move around a lot in all weathers. The lack of exercise and oxygen in winter makes me tired and is also not good for my joints. I especially miss my daily bike ride to the office. The paths were too smooth, there was snow everywhere, the wind was icy, the ten kilometres by bike were too much for me. But I needed exercise to compensate for my sedentary computer work. For me, movement is also a lightning conductor against stress. I sort my thoughts, develop and plan new ideas. So I decided to run twice a week in the evenings, after work, and I was doing well.

To swing into spring with more momentum, I wanted to also fast. Thereby giving my body and mind a break. Spring is very well suited for this. But I could only do it for three days. I felt weak, shaky and cold, and I was in no way able to work. So I ended the fast, and I ate kohlrabi, carrot and apple in the mornings and a fresh grain meal for lunch. After that I felt well again and was satisfied.

We planned to go to a local carnival. When I looked in the mirror, I felt very pale. I noticed that I had got some lighter strands of hair over the winter. Maybe I was wanting to cheat the dull winter when I had an idea to try out a hair dye. I'd never dyed my hair before. As a child I often felt unhappy with my reddish-blond hair, especially since I couldn't avoid the matching summer freckles. Later I was very often asked what my "beautiful colour" was called. And now that the colour is slowly fading, am I missing it? I'd like it back!

Without further ado, I bought a packet of hair dye, read everything thoroughly and put Saturday evening aside to do it. I wasn't particularly worried. I knew that most people dyed their hair regularly, and I thought the application time of 20 minutes was short. I also wanted to reduce the duration of exposure time, as I did not want a strong colour. My body can take it, I thought Just as I had thought previously when applying cosmetics. But I simply had no idea what I was doing. There were also no warnings on the package that would have unsettled me. When it was done, the colour looked a little unusual, but I was happy with the result.

On Sunday morning, however, I was gripped by the sheer horror. After I felt a burning sensation in my lower abdomen, I went to the toilet and saw a lot of blood. I didn't understand how that was possible. What did I eat yesterday? I couldn't think of anything unusual. I hadn't eaten anything sweet, and we hadn't eaten a big roast, it had been mostly my normal vegetables. I couldn't understand what was happening. I hadn't had that in years. Where had it come from all of a sudden? I was completely confused, but I was sure that I could solve the problem with consistent raw food. Ulcerative colitis flares up intermittently. But such a sudden outbreak wasn't possible! Things did not improve during the day. And the next day brought no improvement either. I was getting more and more restless. There must be a reason, a trigger! I washed my hair immediately, thoroughly, several times and for a very long time, in order to remove as much of the dye as possible. I didn't feel better during the day.
On Tuesday I went to the hairdresser and had my very long hair cut. A short hairstyle. The problem did not change! I thought if the dye was removed, all I would need to do is eat raw food, and the inflammation would heal. But that didn't work! After three days there was no change! The problem was probably not the colour in my hair, but the active ingredients that had long since been distributed after two days throughout my body via the scalp and the bloodstream. I didn't want to take the drugs again, as they merely suppress the symptoms. Taking the drugs

wouldn't rid my body of the cause which I suspected was the chemicals from the dye.

Although I had already fasted for a few days, even though I felt helpless, I saw this as the only way to reduce the toxins. I could only endure the fast for two days. I got so dizzy, I couldn't even find rest in bed. My head was spinning, I couldn't remember where I was. I couldn't get up, it was black before my eyes, but I couldn't lie down either. So I started to eat again and hoped to be able to up on my two feet again quickly.

Before I started fasting, I should have consulted a doctor who was experienced in removing toxic substances. Unfortunately, I didn't know anyone. Neither did I know who to contact in order to find a suitable contact.

I was getting worse and worse and didn't know what to do. My sister remembers a phone call: "I'd never seen you like this before, you were completely at the end, you cried and kept saying, I want to come to Haldensleben, I want to see my mum now." The following week Helmut drove me to my parents, who lovingly looked after and cared for me.

I love being with my parents, it feels like a piece of childhood and I feel very safe. The week did me good, I was able to collect my thoughts and gain distance. There was no improvement in the symptoms. But after talking to my parents and sister, I knew I needed to find a doctor who could heal me, a doctor who wasn't just focused on medication.

I need a doctor

I was acquainted with a general practitioner who also had training in homeopathy and TCM (Traditional Chinese Medicine). Her detoxification approach finally convinced me, and after discussing it with Helmut, I decided to accept this alternative. She took a lot of time to talk to me about my illness and my general situation. I got the impression that she was looking for deeper causes. I had acupuncture needles in my face and ears. That was unpleasant, especially as I had to drive home afterwards with the needles on my face. The needles should fall out by themselves. During the treatment she gave me homeopathic beads to take. It was supposed to promote detoxification.

Regarding my health she said that the poison had to come out of my body, but she also said that I was nervously very tense. She prescribed Folsan, Magnerot Classic and Mutaflor® suspension to strengthen me and gently suppress the colitis. During the period of detoxification I should definitely avoid raw food, as it would further weaken my body. I was hoping the detox would be over in a few weeks. My symptoms didn't get any better in the following four weeks. Worse still, rheumatic pain began. I suffered from increasing morning stiffness. It was a whole new experience for me. My wrists and finger joints also hurt. My fingers became swollen and I had to see a rheumatologist because I could no longer work with my hands. I had an injection into my wrist, the effect of which lasted for several weeks. Diagnosis: "seronegative enteropathic arthritis," I was prescribed Azulfidine RA film-coated tablets No. 300. The rheumatologist did not go along with my hunch the hair dye could be the cause of my discomfort. Unfortunately, he couldn't give me any other cause of the disease either. He also questioned my experiences with the healing effects of raw food. I didn't feel understood. I guess that's one reason why I couldn't make up my mind to hand in the prescription. I was afraid of the "medication spiral" that I already knew too well, with so many painful side effects. My hope was still that the toxins would gradually leave my body by themselves and that, as a result, I would slowly get better again.

But the bleeding and pain continued to increase. In June I received cortisone for two weeks at a low dose to calm the colitis. It helped quickly, but immediately after weaning, the rheumatic symptoms continued to worsen.

I now felt empty and exhausted, and my despondency increased. Of course, I also talked to the general practitioner, who I mentioned earlier, about my diet. I described to her how I have been eating in the last few years. She thought that my diet was good and helpful. She also favoured vegetables, but stuck to the fact that I should only eat everything in cooked form. I

should consistently avoid raw foods. She also told me to drink a lot, especially boiled and cooled water, and if I was cold, hot water. I tried to follow these dietary guidelines, as I assumed that this diet would be helpful in conjunction with acupuncture and Chinese and Ayurvedic healing teachings. She also pre-scribed healing clay for me to take, Mutaflor® intestinal bacte-ria, Moviprep powder, and if the bleeding got worse, Salofalk and Budenofalk rectal foam in alternation.
But none of that improved my situation. I was getting worse and worse, and I was getting thinner. I now felt like I had lost the thread of my life forever.

Helplessness

Our youngest daughter Josefine had now also graduated from high school, I was very proud of my independent girls. How can they be so big already, I have already missed so much due to my illness!
In May, the Leavers' Ball was just around the corner. The cele-bration took place in Berlin. It was a very big event, as several classes were involved. Josefine wore a long, copper-coloured ball gown. She is very natural in her ways and hardly ever wears make-up. Before we left, she shook her long, curly hair, brushed it, twisted it upwards without using a mirror, and stuck it in place. It was as simple as that. She was beautiful. Now she was ready to actually go. But it wasn't that easy for me, because I had to "run" all the time, so we couldn't drive. Every time I thought I was ready to leave, I had to go again! We were late and missed the photo shoot. I felt so sorry! Josefine took every-thing in her stride and was very laid back, she even cheered me up. Her priorities weren't photography, they were her mummy. Where did she get that serenity from at her age?
Also in the following weeks there was no ray of hope for my recovery, as much as I hoped, since another family celebration was coming up. My sister and my brother-in-law both turned 50 within a week. My party mood fit into a snail shell. I was

happy when I could manage my normal working days and rested at the weekends. How was I supposed to get through a party? I still weighed 54 kilograms.

So I called my sister. She listened to my problems and promised to step up. I knew she'd find a solution. She organised it so that there would be enough vegetables on the buffet: "There will be plenty of fresh salad, including grated carrots and kohlrabi," she promised.

She knew from the past how important raw food was for me in order to reduce my symptoms. I hadn't told them that I was now supposed to avoid raw food. The most important thing was to ensure my personal "escape route". In the restaurant there were three ladies toilets, one was OUT OF ORDER that evening! For me, of course. Catrin had put a sign on the door and the problem was solved! I had my own "cabin", she assured me.

A bad attack of rheumatism

The rheumatism also continued to worsen. The extent of pain was new to me. It was unbearable, especially in the morning. It was agonising getting myself out of bed and I could only put one foot in front of the other with difficulty. Every single movement I made hurt. Finally I stood up, I started to slowly do move and do relaxation exercises on a gymnastics mat. A dry brushing followed and then a long, warm shower. It was almost noon before I could move quite normally.

Since I did not want to take any medication at first, my doctor prescribed me massages. I was afraid of addiction and feared the resulting spiral of ever-increasing doses, like the devil to holy water, because I also knew how hard it was to get away from it.

In August, sciatica was added to the mix. The pain was immense and I was on all fours on the floor, I had to go to the toilet and couldn't move! I refused an injection because I feared the side effects, instead I rubbed myself with Voltaren gel. Now I had stomach ache, my stomach was on fire, and I curled up even more. I was lying in bed whimpering and couldn't do anything at all. The next day the stomach pain subsided. I tried to get some freedom of movement by doing some gymnastic exercise. I also used my hay flower bag. This is heated in a pot with a sieve over steam and then, still hot, placed on the affected area, in my case that was on my lower back. Like a warm, moist envelope, my body was packaged up, then a long rest period followed. I fell into a deep and sound sleep.

When I woke up, I could move better. Within three days I got a good handle on my back pain. But that wasn't all, because now a strange touch sensitivity began on my body. I was now happy that I refused the injection against sciatica, otherwise I would have thought the new problems were a side effect. Why was I suddenly so sensitive to touch? My arms, thighs and back were affected. Even my clothes touching my body hurt. My doctor diagnosed it as fibromyalgia and prescribed connective tissue massages. This was a relaxing and gentle massage, and I found these moments helpful because my painful body was pampered. However, the fibromyalgia did not disappear afterwards. I strictly adhered to the prescribed dietary rules. I steamed all the vegetables and didn't eat any raw food.

Still no end in sight

At the end of September, my health deteriorated, I was having forty bowel movements a day and twelve at night. In the meantime, when I wasn't sitting on the toilet, I was collapsed in bed for short periods of sleep. I felt drained and exhausted. I hardly ever touched food anymore. My sister said to me: "I thought you were only eating psyllium husks these days!" I moved back into my "safe place" in the basement, right next to the bathroom. For medication, I was taking 3x2 tablets of Salofalk.

I still went to acupuncture regularly because I was still hoping that the desired effect would finally come. I still found the placement of the needles very unpleasant. It made me aggressive and painful at the same time. I can't actually say whether acupuncture has contributed to detoxification. My doctor now developed a detailed diet plan for me and explained the individual items in the context of a nutrition consultation. Their indications were based on Ayurvedic medicine. They consisted mainly of fruit and vegetables, everything was gently cooked. There was little meat and animal protein. Sugar was forbidden, white flour was allowed.

After I had submitted the statement of account to both health insurance companies, I was informed: "The expenses for a diet plan or a nutritional consultation are not part of the insurance cover ...".

Experience teaches good lessons

It was the end of November. I was signed off sick again. I found my condition hopeless. I hadn't been any help in the office for a long time. I felt that I couldn't go on like this, I was completely powerless and felt physically at the end of my tether. I was tormented day and night by my illness and the immense pain.

It was clear to me now that I had to do something myself. Help yourself, because nobody else will. I have to trust in what helped me back then, many years ago. I am will exclusively and consistently fall back on my personal nutritional experiences. From this point forward, I put the fresh grain dish back on my daily menu: Raw grain, fresh fruit and organic cream. I started slowly, with small portions. And honestly, my body seemed to want to stabilise in the days that followed. I also ate pure raw food: apple, carrot and kohlrabi, several times a day. I stopped eating boiled food. Within the next two weeks I was slowly getting better. Every day I felt the decreasing bowel movements and the relaxation. I expanded the range of vegetables I ate daily. I tolerated the vegetables well, I didn't notice any problems. There must be people who find this more difficult; it worked very well for me.

Since I was on sick leave, a representative of the health insurance company came to visit me. In order to speed up my recovery, he recommended that I apply to the German Pension Insurance Union for rehabilitation. It would be very straightforward, he said. "Will rehab change anything, are there any other treatments?" I asked myself. It gave me hope, because I wanted to support the healing with all possible means.

Helmut also liked the idea and thought that I should definitely give it a go. After all, they may have dedicated doctors with more experience, specialists even. It's important that I get well again, nothing else matters, he said, immediately dispelling my concerns. In my application to the German Pension Insurance Union I was able to suggest a clinic myself. I wrote to the DCCV (Deutsche Morbus Crohn Colitis ulcerosa Vereinigung DCCV e.V. The federal association for chronic inflammatory diseases of the digestive tract) asking about recommended clinics for my disease and was immediately sent an extensive list.
Based on this, I started to gather more information from the Internet. What was important to me? I was looking for a clinic with a focus on nutrition in ulcerative colitis. A diet that strengthens the immune system, is rich in vital substances and is nutritious. For me, this also included cookery courses and information about foods to avoid. After my rheumatism over the last months, it was important to me that the focus of the clinic was also on the treatment of rheumatic symptoms. I wanted to have good physiotherapy treatments such as massages or exercise therapy. And of course I also wanted to improve my general health and strengthen my body; I consider sports such as hiking, gymnastics and swimming to be ideal for this. In addition, I would like to learn biofeedback or other relaxation techniques professionally. I had so many desires and dreams!
I was particularly interested in alternative healing methods, such as naturopathy, herbalism or Kneipp therapies. I also wanted to learn how to prevent the disease in the future. Are there any particular things that colitis patients should be aware of in their lives?
I hoped to obtain a lot of new information, through lectures as well as through discussions with other patients. That is a lot

of wishes, but at the end of the day, the rehab needed to be a success for me.

At first glance, my search resulted in many appealing websites. Unfortunately, I didn't find the information I was looking for. The clinic websites are in no way conclusive when it came to answering my questions. I didn't learn anything about the philosophy of the clinics. There was no information about the courses and services on offer or even about the type of food. Patient opinions and evaluations in forums also didn't provide any further helpful information either. I had to assume that not everything was written on the website and in the end I decided, more with hope than with any actual knowledge, on a clinic in Bad Brückenau. I would have preferred a clinic that was close to me, since a long train ride was unimaginable for me at this time. So, filled with confidence, I sent in my documents and hoped that if I was accepted in a few weeks' time, I would be able to start this journey. The rehab was approved after a week, so before Christmas. But I wasn't

"fit to travel," so I asked for a postponement until January. The postponement was approved.

But by the middle of December I felt much better. I was amazed how well the raw food took effect now. Every day I ate salads made of raw turnips, lettuce, cucumbers and apples. My bleeding decreased daily and my body calmed down. By Christmas I was completely pain-free. The bleeding had stopped, and I could omit the first Salofalk tablet. My fibromyalgia symptoms also disappeared. The morning stiffness almost completely petered out over the New Year period. The clear and, as I was astonished to notice, now very rapid improvement in the illness, made me relax me and took away my worries before the trip in January. With now just five to eight stools a day, mostly in the morning, I was able to make the journey. I even felt so stable that I began to look forward to the journey. I was so hopeful about all the new things I would now learn about my disease. I'll never let my body go through that again. By the end of the year, I dropped off another tablet of Salofalk.

Had my body needed such a long time to detoxify? Would it have been more successful had I have eaten a consistent raw diet the whole time? Or would there have been some other way to detoxify my body in order for it to regain its own balance? These questions concerned me. Are there people affected who have experienced similar problems? I was hoping to learn all about it during rehab!

Medication costs in 2006: 484,80 Euro

2007

Rehab as an opportunity

For medication, I take 3x1 tablet of Salofalk, psyllium husks (seeds of the sand plantain, stimulate bowel movements as a bulk-forming agent) and magnesium for the cramps. I have had very good experiences with psyllium husks.
In early January, I went to Bad Brückenau. I decided to find rehabilitation companions with a positive attitude to life and who didn't talk so much about illnesses. I wanted active, humorous people who spread happiness. My expectations were met immediately.
At the bus stop from Fulda to Bad Brückenau I met Waltraut from Kassel. We hit it off straight away. I immediately noticed that Waltraut was very open-minded and had a sense of humour. We had double the luck, because we found ourselves at the same table in the clinic. She had undergone colorectal cancer surgery and by all accounts was ready to face life again. The reasons for the rehab were very different at our table. I was very saddened by the fate of a 22-year old young girl. She had Crohn's disease, and the result of many operations meant that she was left with only 1.5 metres of small intestine. She had undergone several intestinal surgeries since her childhood, yet she is a cheerful, curly blonde ray of sunshine! Apart from me, another patient suffered from ulcerative colitis; he was severely affected by the disease. He had had hardly any periods of remission in his recovery, but he hadn't suffered from the severe flare-ups that I knew. This was the first time I had had the opportunity to exchange experiences with other people affected by the disease.
Life in a clinic like this has its own rules. I received a weekly plan and found out which therapies were intended for me and

which of my personal wishes could be taken into account. First I wanted to take a look at everything and get used to it. It was a good thing that I already knew Waltraut, because in our free time we did a lot together. We went hiking, played table tennis, listened to music, talked or just stayed quiet.

Unfulfilled wishes

As I mentioned, I came to this rehabilitation clinic with great expectations, and it quickly became clear that many things would not be met. The most important topic to me was nutrition. What does this look like for people with a weak immune system? According to Dr. Bruker, nutrition is meant to stabilise the immune system, reinforce self-healing powers and strengthen the body. A nutritious and wholesome diet rich in vital substances with a lot of raw food is the best way to do this. The daily meals offered here were in no way consistent with these findings. At mealtimes, you had to be particularly quick to get your fair share of any salad and vegetables. I also don't like an evening meal with brown bread, cooked sausage and cheese slices. Genuine, good wholemeal bread and fresh salad would be much tastier. Lunch dishes were mostly soft boiled, often bland and tasteless. Herbs and spices were not given any importance in the kitchen. During a conversation with the doctor, I was told that most patients had undergone major surgery and suffered from various digestive problems. Only a low-fibre diet ensures that everyone can tolerate the food, and that's hard enough for many. When I told him that I was used to a different diet, which was very good for me, He simply recommended that I eat the available raw food and that that would be sufficient. I couldn't understand why an individual meal plan couldn't be arranged. That's why I had subdued expectations when I went on the cookery course run by a trained nutritionist. As suspected, I was disappointed. The main topic here was also a low-fibre diet. My questions about fresh food and wholemeal were pushed aside as inappropriate. Diarrhoea, painful flatulence, spasmodic pain can be the result of eating raw food, I was told.

On this course we prepared a menu consisting of salad, soup and a main course, in this case: "Fish on a bed of vegetables with herb sauce". The vegetables were gently cooked and then put back into the oven with the fish. This was supposed to make the fish tastier, but unfortunately the vegetables were no longer firm to the bite. This was seen as a positive thing in the context of a low-fibre diet. The recommendation of finishing off the dish in the microwave shocked me! There was no fresh fruit. Boiled fruit for dessert contains too much sugar. How was I supposed to deal with that? This cookery course did not correspond in any way to what I had hoped to gain in terms of knowledge. There was no information on how to restrict sugar, exchange superfine flours for wholemeal flours or avoid industrially processed foods containing artificial additives. On the contrary: sugar, sweeteners, flour, starch, margarine, low-fat dairy products and processed cheese were even part of the course recipes. I was very disappointed! Nutrition is the most important basis for strengthening the immune system, and thus my health. I couldn't believe that this fact didn't matter at the clinic.

I also wanted information on medicinal herbs, wild fruits or spices that are good for the intestines. A herbal or wild fruit hike that teaches you about important active ingredients, what belongs in a hay flower pillow and how to use it would've fit the concept well. There was no information or discussion about artificial additives and pollutants in food, cosmetics and the environment. When I finally got an opportunity to ask questions at an event, the subject was dismissed as being not of general interest. I was examined for lactose intolerance and I was found not to have a problem.

The activities on offer for improving physical strength included aqua aerobics, fitness and walking. I liked the aqua aerobics very much, because the joints were spared yet at the same time the muscles were getting a workout, which did me good. I could

also imagine regularly doing aqua aerobics after rehabilitation.
I could see this as a preventative measure against my neck and
hand symptoms as well. Is there a sports club for aqua aerobics?
In front of the swimming pool, there was a Kneipp pool for
treading water, which I used daily and extensively. Since I moved
a lot, I quickly warmed up afterwards.
I had lost a lot of weight over the last few months, but what
was worse was that my muscles had fallen by the wayside. So, I
regularly used the available dates in the gym. I did everything,
tried to do my best and to do the exercises to strengthen my
arms and back with more success each day, but it was very difficult for me, and I found it very depressing when I saw how
easy it was for others to do the exercises. I felt like my body was
so much older than I actually was.

From my previous experience I knew that biofeedback does me
good. The clinic offered progressive muscle relaxation and
biofeedback. I wanted to register for both courses. Unfortunately, there wasn't enough capacity so I could only take the
progressive muscle relaxation course. Massages were not part
of the healing programme. It was explained to me, when I
asked, that the deletion was for cost-saving reasons. This was
not mentioned on the clinic's website. Unfortunately, the clinic
also provided no details on current services before the start of
the rehabilitation.
After my extensive rheumatic symptoms over last few months,
I felt this to be a particularly great disappointment. But there
were spas, and I always looked forward to them! It is a wonderful feeling when the bath is already sunken! I got a headrest
and had twenty minutes of peace. It was particularly nice not
having to take care of yourself!

The very kind pampering by the caregivers, my cheerful, open-
minded fellow-spa-goers and the complete freedom from stress
did me good and led to me feeling stronger and having a better
sense of well-being. Yet, I have to say, I didn't receive any answers to my questions or any professional advice on self-help. I
decided to communicate this to the pension insurance union.

When I got back home, trouble was waiting for me: it was my health insurance representative who had recommended that I apply for rehabilitation with the German Pension Insurance. That's why I didn't get sick pay for the period I was in rehab. The reason being that I only receive sickness benefit if I attend rehab at an institution chosen by my health insurance company. What's the reasoning for this? I realised that I hadn't been sufficiently informed about this option before. It didn't occur to me that there were such facilities available. I hadn't found anything out about them in the glossy customer magazines produced by the health insurance company. Nor was I informed about this option by the representative either. Why not?

Help yourself because nobody else will

I need to take better care of myself. Especially when it's a question of convenience and I start putting things off because I don't have the time! Habits play a big role, they form without us even being aware of them. To recognise something as wrong is one thing, to change what has been recognised is much more difficult. I just can't simply change who I am and will have to learn to struggle through!
I mustn't look at others and think what's good for them is good for me too. It really isn't. I'm different, I'm more sensitive, more fragile, more vulnerable, and that's why I have this disease. I have to keep that in mind, only then will I be able to do it.

In the book: "Liver, bile, gastrointestinal and pancreatic diseases" by Dr. M. O. Bruker (19th edition 2001), it also reads as follows:

"... It therefore requires the guidance of a doctor who is experienced in nutritional issues, who assures the patient, accompanies him over a long period of time and helps him to overcome crises."

I'd like more doctors who can do this. Doctors who not only prescribe, but heal. I would particularly like to emphasise the following sentence:

"Relapses occur frequently because the patient no longer adheres so strictly to the dietary guidelines as a result of improvement. ..."

I've experienced this time and time again. And yet after a while everything seems to be blown away by the wind! Why is that so hard? Do I not trust myself enough?!

My new routine

I immediately started to do what I had planned and registered at a gym. My experience from rehab has shown me that I still have a lot to do to get fit again. Good muscles also strengthen the immune system. In the gym I was offered a Tai Chi course. I was curious about it, so signed up right away. Tai Chi is very versatile, it is used for relaxation and composure, is a good school of balance and promotes concentration. Tai Chi is a martial art, in which the energy of an
"opponent" is absorbed and used for self-defence. This involves slow, soft-flowing movements that correspond to the natural movement pattern of the joints. At the beginning, however, I had to learn to leave my work pace at the door and to find my body's own natural energy flow. I can almost always switch off when creating these figures and shapes.
The application to my health insurance company for a cost contribution for regular visits to a gym, back physiotherapy or the Tai Chi course was rejected. I was also refused attendance to an aqua aerobics course over several weeks on the grounds that only individual treatments, no group therapies, are paid for.
I think it is more important to invest in good disease prevention than in medication, because that is real health care. But unfortunately my opinion is not at issue here.

I had already stopped taking the last of my medication during rehab. Although I felt good, I didn't feel as euphoric and happy as I did back then. It may have been related to the discontinuation of the Imurek at the time. My further recovery was not a runaway success either, I had to drive and motivate myself every day. But as the weeks go on, I do feel more and more that it is worth it!

I go to the gym three times a week now. Not because I dream of a super body but because I want to build up sufficient muscle to feel well, no more neck tensions and no more back pain. I put my fitness routine together in such a way that all muscle groups get some work, but so that I only use my strength moderately. Afterwards I would enjoy a relaxing sauna and cycle back to the office, feeling fresh, lively and invigorated.

I can also manage my daily commute to work by bike again. It was hard for me at first. But now I'm proud to be back on track. The nine kilometres make me feel better in the morning and allow me switch off better in the evening. However, it wasn't until summer arrived that I truly felt like my body was my own again.

True to the old adage: "There's no such thing as bad weather, just the wrong clothing" I kept on with my daily bike rides until the end of November. This is an important daily challenge for me, because mentally it also makes me feel much more balanced.

Of course, a daily bike ride would have also done Helmut good. But we always needed a car outside the office to be safe. He allowed me cycle and let me go and do sports several times a week. He was happy that I was well again and supported me in everything I do! I'm really very lucky with my dear husband!

This renewed experience of illness has changed a lot in my life. I now enjoy many more things and approach things more slowly and with greater composure. Happiness lies in enjoying things. I now take time to regularly paint again. One evening a week is devoted to my art group, which also runs when I can't be there. For me this is relaxing, as it often relieves me of the time pressure that I can now no longer deal with. The excessive demands of work and illness over this last year has left traces that still limit my ability to work under pressure.

Inline skating – it conjures up images of technique and speed – and it's a great experience. The newly developed Fläming-Skate® is a perfect for this sport. Smooth asphalt paths stretching over 300 kilometres meander through a beautiful and sparsely populated area in the south of the Teltow-Fläming district. They cross forests, meadows, fields and small villages. We seized this opportunity with growing enthusiasm. We regularly arranged evening or day trips with the children or friends. There are several small stretches of twelve kilometres. I enjoy the fast movement, which places demands on the whole body, but still allows you to talk and enjoy the surroundings and the weather. The longest distance that I skated was 56 kilometres with a friend this summer. I'm so pleased that my body is finally able to do this again.

Feel, see, smell, taste …

Training to become a health consultant in Lahnstein is something that I just can't get out of my mind. The knowledge and experience could help me to become more confident in my cooking and lifestyle. I always bugs me when I realise that my health is a "side job". The contacts and the exchange with like-minded people with similar problems would be a great support. But I have no idea how I can do this alongside my work; as much as I would like to do it, at the moment, unfortunately, I see no way of putting this project into practice.

Oliver, Helmut's younger son, has lived with us for several years. He does a lot of sports, is health conscious and as such is very interested in my diet. In the daily cooking chores, we share the preparation of the food. At 30 years of age, he has a good appetite, so the portions he prepares tend to be slightly larger.

The fresh grain meal in the morning is an Olympic team effort. When he comes home from doing his sport in the evening – after thoroughly sharpening his knives – a major operation on the salad front follows. Then we cook a vegetable dish with pasta, rice or potatoes. When Helmut comes home late from the office, the table is already set.

I want to learn to bake bread because I want to know what is in my bread and I want to eat bread that I like! I hate the laborious search for good bread and the disappointment I feel when the staff at the bakery do not have sufficient information on the proportion of wholemeal flour and additives in the bread. I don't have the experience. A baking course would be something that would help me now. But who offers a full baking course near me? My search has so far been futile. So I'll just start and gather my own experience.
During this training several stirrers met their maker in the heavy bread dough. My two men have now purchased a kneading machine with a three-litre stainless steel bowl and a more powerful motor. This makes the work easier and less time consuming.
I want sourdough to be the basis for my bread. I had collected various recipes. But they were very different, so I started very carefully to learn the rules of the game when it came to increasing the bacteria.
Good bread requires three things: flour, water and salt. When I grind grain, I get flour, I add water, I get a more or less liquid porridge depending on the quantity. How do I find the right temperature and time? My dear biology and chemistry teacher came to my aid. Since he also loves good bread, I was able to drum up his enthusiasm for my project, especially since baking for two is more fun! He succeeded easily in motivating bacteria that were not visible to us to process our grain porridge into sourdough.
The first loaves were already quite good, and with each new attempt we learnt something new. We are now trying to get the right feel for the processing and rising times. We bake more regularly, and the breads are tastier due to the experience we have gained.

I have adapted what I buy and my inventory to my diet. Of the 25,000 items from the supermarket, I need very little. These essentially include: Vegetables and fruit, salads, herbs, oils, cream, butter, honey, grain, nuts, kernels, seeds, wholemeal rice, wholemeal pasta and also eggs and a little cheese.

I prepare a lot of things myself: I cook jams and fruit purée without sugar or with some honey and apple pectin. Because I have a high yield of fruits, especially raspberries and blueberries, I freeze these in portions. Lushly growing herbs from my garden are chopped, put into oil, frozen or dried, depending on how they taste best to me. I also collect many herbs, flowers and leaves for tea over the summer, which I dry: blackberry leaves, lime blossoms, peppermint, mallow blossoms, rose hips and lemon balm. Our first homemade sauerkraut was a special experience. There was enough for the whole winter and it was used in salads, casseroles, cakes, soups or spicy vegetable casseroles.

Vegetables such as beans, tomatoes, peppers and onions can also be pickled. It's not much work. Cooking will always be an enjoyable voyage of discovery for me – I want to feel, see, smell, taste – I love it!

Beautiful perfect world

The magical world of advertising can no longer tempt me to eat something that my senses don't recognise. In this world, families live in their sweet idyll and are happy about crispy sausages, creamy cheese or look expectantly into a beautifully curved, steaming soup tureen. Who wouldn't want to feel that happy and be a part of it? It creates suspense: inside this steaming soup tureen there can only be something wonderful, you can literally smell it: Soup from a colourful packet. We are used to accepting the hypocrisy of these images but usually know better in our minds. Because when you take a closer look, you wonder: what's actually in the packet? Cheap fat, lots of sugar, salt, flavour enhancers, colourings, and what do the many E numbers actually mean?

Take a clear vegetable soup, for example. Put some of the contents of the bag on your hand. How does the powder feel between your fingers? Look, smell and taste it. You'll feel salt and maybe some meat or Maggi seasoning. But this has nothing to do with vegetables from the garden. When I think of vegetable soup, I think of my grandmother's garden, what a variety there was, beans, onions, kohlrabi, carrots, celery, as well as many herbs and flowers, asters, vetches, snapdragons and roses. In the soup, you'll find a little bit of dried vegetables at the most. When I look at the back of the box, I don't understand most of the ingredients, even my grandmother, who was a perfect cook, couldn't, I'm sure! Because it has nothing to do with her garden.

Flavour enhancers and artificial flavours lead my body to believe it is getting food, which the meal then doesn't deliver. You don't feel full and the artificial flavours lead to the desire for more. In many cases the result is obesity with the resulting symptoms.

When our natural health protection is therefore undermined, common sense is needed. You should therefore avoid food whose original ingredients are no longer recognisable.

Hans-Ulrich Grimm writes in his book "The Soup Lies": "Taste is not a matter of taste, but a message." We need to learn to understand that message again, and this is exactly what a natural diet helps us to do.

Warning signals that help me

It has happened twice in the last few months. My bowel didn't forewarn me but instead sprang a surprise on me.

In both cases, I ate something the evening before at an event that I had already suspected I shouldn't have done. I didn't want to resist the temptation. It wasn't much, I just wanted a taste. But why do I have to taste something if I already suspect that it is not good for me? Why don't I listen to my inner voice in these situations? It was the catering buffet at an event with breaded

Asian fried "things" that I couldn't even describe exactly. I couldn't identify the taste either. About twelve hours later, my bowel reacted with a fine red blood trail.

Fortunately, it disappeared as quickly as it had come. But the shock was deep, the memory of the consequences of dyeing my hair immediately came to mind. I was not in pain, I only saw this one sign, an error message so to speak! Since I had not deviated from my diet in any other way, it remained just a sign.

But the warning was clear. I wasn't careful enough with myself! Through these experiences, I am becoming more and more aware of signals, because it helps me to know my limits. If I'm not sure what I can eat, I'd rather not eat. Nobody starves to death if they skip one or two meals, and if I'm unsure what to expect at an event where there is a buffet, I take an apple, a carrot or a wholemeal roll with me. It's no hassle, and I'm independent. And meanwhile I like to take my criticisms to the event organisers, stating that a modern buffet should include salads of raw food and fruit!

If I have a lot of stress over a long period of time, I notice that I get dry eyes. That is serious evidence that my immune system is suffering and that all mucous membranes, including those in my intestines, may be affected. That's a signal to me now. I have to change my work routine IMMEDIATELY.

Body signals have a function. It is important to get to know what they are and to keep an eye on them: headaches, flatulence, muscle pain, joint stiffness, bleeding – our body seeks dialogue. It always means: watch closely, listen and be loving with yourself. Don't put it off, but take a break NOW!

Medication costs in 2007: 259.00 Euro.

2008

Taking a break

A car stops driving when the tank is empty. Why don't I stick to that rule, too? I need a routine that allows me to refuel regularly. For this I do Tai Chi and Qi Gong in addition to my biofeedback. I like the slow pace at which the exercises are carried out. This peace must come from within, and that can be learned. After exercising, I feel relaxed.

It's also very practical: To place everything aside for a few minutes and look out the window into the distance. Just simply do nothing. I combine this with eye training. A change in focusing at different distances, slowly tracing the treetops with my eyes or the tracking a flight of birds, all of this has a relaxing effect on my stressed eyes.

Raw food days are now also a proven means of well-being for me. For a whole day, I eat only raw vegetables and fruit: kohlrabi, carrots, cauliflower, apples, bananas, the fresh grain dish at noon and a salad in the evening. I only drink water with it. I eat my fill at every meal and treat myself to a little more rest on these days. I feel wonderful on it. The statement: "Raw food is health food" by Dr. Bruker has proved true for me.

Can I eat in restaurants?

Basically, yes. But there are a few criteria the restaurant has to meet for me to make the decision. The most important thing is that the dishes are as natural as possible. I can often tell from the menu. Glancing at other guests' plates is also very helpful. If the menus don't give enough information about the preparation and my imagination isn't enough, I talk to the staff about the dishes before ordering. I have learned to ask questions: What is it? What's in it? Or even: Would you cook this for me like this? For example, I may ask for half a portion and request that the additional portion be served as raw food. Or I could ask if I could get jacket potatoes instead of boiled potatoes. Of course, this is not possible if the potatoes have already been delivered industrially peeled. My meal ALWAYS starts with a large portion of salad, even in restaurants. Then I'll feel stable enough to eat a freshly made pizza, if I have an appetite for it. When we go out for dinner as a couple, each orders their own large plate of salad, and then we often choose one hot dish with two forks.

In my favourite restaurants, in the countryside, you can look into the pots, and even better if the restaurants have their own vegetable garden, this gives me confidence.

If I am at a business event, I check whether there is enough raw food on the buffet. If not, I'm concerned. But if I am able to put together a plate of fresh raw food, then everything else is not a problem.

Thick sauces, fried, breaded, cooked, many desserts, unnaturally colourful things – I generally avoid these things, because I have had bad experiences with them all too often.

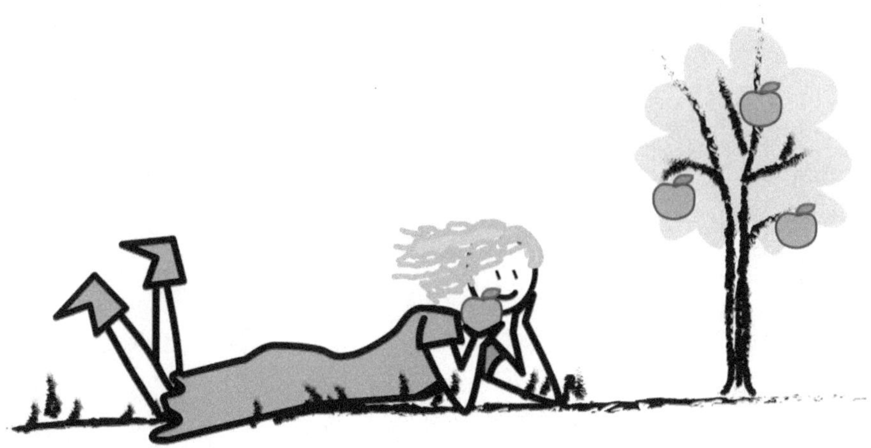

A much harder way

I keep regular e-mail contact with my friend Waltraut, who I met at the rehab. She had apparently defeated cancer after her intestinal surgery and rehab. She was looking forward to her job, which she was going to start again for a few hours at a time. After only a few weeks, however, she was no longer able to cope with the workload and was completely exhausted. The cancer had returned with numerous metastases in the lymph nodes, lungs and liver. Doctors fighting cancer now alternate 14 days of chemotherapy and antibody therapy. As I now know, this can go on for years. Waltraut was very brave during the treatment, although she was very ill and wrote to me about how she used the breaks to lead a normal life. She went on many excursions with her husband or friends. In the hope of recovery, she accepted the side effects of antibody therapy, such as severely inflamed toes, fingers and also the scalp. She never complained. I looked forward to each new letter, because then I knew she was doing well. And even greater was the joy when she came to visit me for a day in the summer and we could finally meet up and hug each other again. We spent a nice day together, chatting about everything and anything.

Medication costs in 2008: 0 Euro.

2009

2240 Kilometres

My 22-year-old bicycle is gone. Maybe it has found a new friend; who knows? It wasn't there when I got off the bus. After such a long time it was very sad for me, because it was as old as my youngest daughter, Josefine. That was my immediate thought. Bicycle thieves don't think about such things, of course.

Since I wanted to cycle a larger radius, I was now looking for a touring bike with a modern gear shift and saddlebags. I was lucky: in a small Potsdam bike shop, I found a wonderful diamond ladies' bike, with a well-sprung leather saddle, a comfortable touring bike with gear hub and nine gears, copper-coloured and beautiful. There also had to be an odometer because I was curious to see whether I would ride as much as I had planned to give my car a rest this year.

In May, I immediately planned my first major bike tour together with my friend, Ellen. We looked for suitable accommodation over the Internet and drove north from Berlin with the Regio. The Berlin-Brandenburg ticket extended to Müritz, the largest lake in Mecklenburg. Anyone who has ever been lucky enough to visit the Mecklenburg Lake District knows what I am writing about. This region is a paradise for cyclists, as well as for those who love bathing, canoeing and kayaking. The weather was still very fresh, but we had the right clothes in our luggage. The cycle path around Müritz was around 80 kilometres, we enjoyed the first forty kilometres very much and took it easy, because it was wonderful sunny day. Then it slowly became dark and began to rain heavily. Conveniently, there is a bus with a bike trailer that "collects" drifters like us, but this only travelled on the side of the lake that we already been on! The same way back, by bus, we agreed, was absolutely not what we wanted. We reached Waren with some effort, but without any hardship, and were happy. When I got back home, I knew: I wanted more of this!

Our children were grown up, and had flown the nest. For us parents this means that we can and may plan our free time differently. It was the same for my sister. In June, I wanted to go cycling with her for a few days.
The Havelland region was our destination. This is a fantastically beautiful area and lies in the middle of nowhere. Small villages, wide fields and meadows. There are no hills or mountains – it's simply the Havelland for as far as the eye can see. If you see white sails gliding over green meadows, then the River Havel is not far. It is pure relaxation. In the Westhavelland nature park it is quite dark. This region is so sparsely populated that stargazers come here to enjoy it because it is the darkest place in Germany.
We found quarters in a romantic farm in Barnewitz. There was even wholefood cuisine here, which we enjoyed with a cheerful, relaxed family.

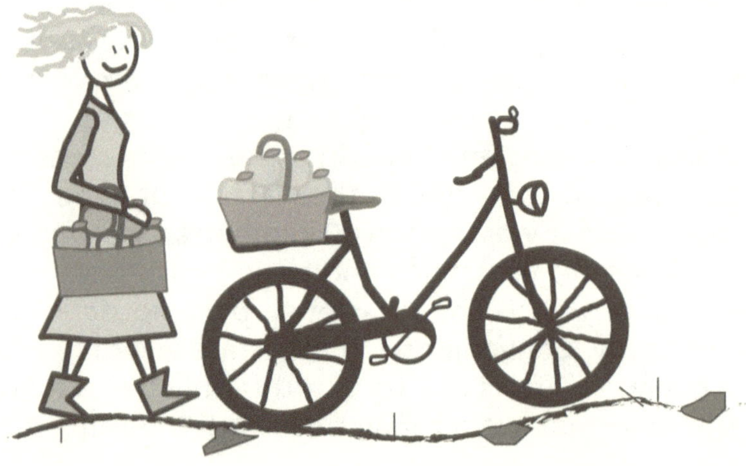

A sisters' holiday is a wonderful thing. It gave us the chance, since we are both self-employed, to spend a lot of time together and to talk to each other. Memories from childhood were awakened and dreams for the future exchanged.

Cycling tours are addictive! I'm rediscovering my home. Because when you travel the road by bike, you see much more than you do from the car. Remote villages and farmsteads, deep forests, quiet nature parks or narrow bridges offer a completely different picture of the landscape. But do you know a region if you know the landscape? I don't think so. People and their way of life are just as much a part of it, and that too is much more pleasant by bike; the friendly greetings are second nature when you enter a village. And since cycling whets my appetite and I love cooking, I started looking for what was growing in my region and what is traditionally sizzling in the kitchens. Out of curiosity, I stopped by the farmers' shops en route. Here I learnt what was currently maturing, how it's cultivated, fertilised and harvested. You can try-and-buy right away. The fact that the vegetables here were not as uniform as in the supermarket was no problem for me. On the contrary: each piece is unique. Curved cucumbers, twisted turnips, tomatoes with noses, twin plums or triple cherries taste just as good or better than their European standard siblings. Taking the fruits as they grow is wonderful and I am more than pleased to make such discoveries. I arrange my purchases in my basket without rustling bags, so that it is a pleasure to look at them.
Tips on processing, a few recipes and fresh trip rations were also picked up en route. A bowl of cherries fitted into my bike bag and gave me a burst of energy! The juicy, plump cherries are a fireworks display for connoisseurs – from the sweet juice to the enthusiastic spitting out of the stone.
There are many traditions and festivals in my region that are increasingly being cultivated. Village and local history museums, mills and village churches are included in them. At these events you can learn a lot about village traditions, old cultivation techniques or farmers' cooking habits. I tried how delicious, cold butter tastes straight from the wooden barrel and I was pleased

to see ceramic pots with holes for the production of curd cheese from raw milk. I also got to know the old tradition of baking Klemmkuchen, a type of griddle cake, on an open fire. In the villages there are village ovens, which are fired up for the festivals. In doing so, old baking traditions are revived.

What always impresses me about traditional cuisine is that a variety of dishes are created with just a few fresh ingredients. The quality of the ingredients and especially the flair of the cook is of imperative, resulting in many local variations of one and the same recipe.

When the cycling season was coming to an end, I had racked up 2240 kilometres on my odometer. This was such a great success for me!

Snoopy is also sick

It was autumn and I was worried because our dog, Snoopy, seemed more and more exhausted as the days went by. Was it joint problems or just the fact that he was getting older? He was now nine years old; and he wanted to walk but couldn't make the long distance, alongside my bike, to the office. So we arranged for Helmut to pick him up by car on the way. I got off the bike, walked at his pace and talked to him, but it hurt me so much to see his strength diminish.

One morning his entire body was trembling, he didn't want to lie down. Josefine was just at home for a few days, and we could rely on her to take care of him, so we went to the office. It didn't get any better, and when she tried to take him to the vet's, he collapsed in front of her car. She lifted him in and drove to the vet's. It was an eleventh-hour rescue! He had a reticulated tumour in his stomach and had suffered an intestinal rupture. The vet operated immediately.

After the operation, he had to stay at the veterinary clinic. Since Josefine had only this weekend off, she couldn't say goodbye to him. She didn't know if he'd make it, if she'd ever see him again. That was particularly difficult for Josefine. After her big sister had moved to Berlin and she was usually alone due to our long working day, Snoopy became her most loyal companion. My heart ached because I knew how much she was suffering because of his illness.

When we were able to pick him up after an endless week, he was very weak and upset. He had a 30-centimetre-long wound on his stomach that was still very weepy. Animals want to lick their wounds. This is a great disinfectant, but can also lead to the reopening of incompletely healed wounds. So, he was given a large lampshade collar. This hindered him not only in seeing but also in eating. The smell of home quickly calmed him down. But the thing around his neck was bothering him. His constant attempts to get rid of this unpopular neck ruff by whatever means necessary over the next few weeks led to some extremely funny situations. Food that was appropriate to his breed and close attention had a positive effect on the healing process. After only four weeks, the wound had healed to such an extent that we were able to remove the collar. Rolling and running through the grass showed just how happy he was to have his freedom back.

Medication costs in 2009: 0 Euro.

2010

Nutritious catering and cyclists' sandwiches

In January we went to the Baltic Sea for a week's holiday. Snoopy had recovered well in the meantime, and it was nice for all of us to experience him walking through the sand adventurously, getting up to all kinds of mischief and feeling visibly comfortable.
By spring he could walk next to my bike to the office every day again.

In February I'll be 50 years old – a new feeling, but I think I'm okay with it. It's something very adult, something special, that's what's going through my mind. Finally, we've been grandparents for some time now. Helmut's eldest son has two children and being grandma and grandpa to them brings us so much joy. My darling husband and the children organised a great party for me; together with my parents, siblings and all my friends. This didn't take place in a restaurant, instead we rented a room in a square barn, which had been completely restored. It was a rustic ambience with a complete kitchen. I wanted to prepare the buffet for 50 people myself with my girls! Of course, in line with my new cooking habits, so mostly whole foods. We tried different recipes and changed them according to the fresh ingredients available to us. Our buffet included colourful salads, warm vegetables and wholesome pasta dishes, vegetable finger food and, of course, a sweet dessert. We were under a lot of time pressure the whole day, but still it was the funniest kitchen day I have ever experienced, it was a pure party atmosphere. My happy girls thought so too. Everything went according to plan and my young ladies surprised me with their refreshing ideas.

When everything was packed and stowed in the car, we were worried that there wouldn't be enough food. After all, we had never cooked for so many guests!
How do you gauge whether a meal was good or not? You ask the guests. And they were very enthusiastic, everyone wanted to taste everything. At the end there was almost nothing left. It was worth all the daring and experimenting. Besides the beautiful celebration, it was a wonderful experience. I had no idea that this had triggered a new idea in the long run.

Cycling for the soul

I wanted to go on another 3-day bike trip to the Havelland in spring with my sister. In Paretz an der Havel, we also found a host who put a lot of effort into fulfilling our dietary wishes.
We drove through Potsdam, without any worries, past "sans souci", into the lovely landscape between the Havel lakes. Prussian kings had once created their summer residences here. Rock formations, lakes, watercourses, meadows, grasslands and forests alternated. By bike, you can combine the enjoyment of nature and physical training with a truly cultural experience. That was also our objective.
Having just arrived, we went on a voyage of discovery. Here, in Paretz, where King Friedrich Wilhelm III of Prussia and his wife Queen Luise once used Paretz Castle as their summer residence, there was much to see. Thanks to the "Charlotte" cable ferry, we could also "change sides" without any problems. After crossing the River Havel, the Havel cycle path leads either to Potsdam or to the city of Brandenburg.
At the end of our rides, our childhood memories once again brought charm to these days. We opened up our "treasure trove of childhood memories" and chatted a lot about them. My sister recalls things from our childhood completely differently to me. Talking about it helps us both to understand our childhood better. Even the feeling I had as a child that my brother Uli had so many advantages over me. Today I realise

that it wasn't easy for him either with two older sisters. Because as the only boy, he didn't have a close playmate who was interested in the same things like we older girls did.

I love to just walk out of the house and start cycling, in flat Brandenburg there were no hills to stop me. Sometimes we would put our bikes on the car and drive a bit further into the countryside, into the Spreewald, the Oderland or Fläming.
It makes me feel good when I can cycle the daily route to work in almost any weather. It clears my head and gives my body, which gets stressed through sitting down, the opportunity to work out a little. I find cycling stimulating and refreshing. It falls in line with my current attitude to life – to use more energy or just let my thoughts roll in my mind. This is how ideas are born. It's similar with the inline skating, the wind seems to sweep everything out of my body that doesn't belong in there. And at the same time, my thoughts become free. I feel strengthened by the intensive movement of my body and feel reborn afterwards! Together with my friend, I even set a new inline skating daily record of 65 kilometres this year.

In order to replenish my rapidly diminishing energy reserves while cycling, I was looking for a workable solution. What could be better than a good wholemeal roll on which you can chew, perchance to dream awhile at your leisure? But where could I find a bread roll like that? I'll bake it myself, I decided. A wheat sourdough would be most suitable for this. However, Brandenburg is a rye county, which is why a third of rye is added to the fine sourdough. The whole thing will be an energy bomb with a large portion of roughly chopped dried fruit and a handful of hazelnuts. The rolls will be stick-shaped, so they fit into my handlebar bag; because of the sourdough they don't dry out so quickly and give a lot of energy if you chew on them slowly while cycling.

Pure nature

At harvest time, we go to pick our own fruit in fruit yards, a large number of which are located around Berlin. Even if the Mark Brandenburg is affectionately and rather mockingly referred to as "the sandbox of the Holy Roman Empire", there is more than just sand, pines, birches and heather. The fruit growers offer strawberries, cherries, raspberries, blueberries, apples or plums for self-harvesting. We nibble until our bellies are rounded, and nothing else will fit in. We don't rest, but we fill the baskets and boxes with the most wonderful fruits. A life just like in the land of milk and honey. The fee we pay is appropriate and takes any berries that may have fallen into our mouths along the way into account. The treats are stored or frozen at home.

Seeing where my food comes from is becoming more and more important to me now. I enjoy that I can increasingly determine that myself. I love the natural taste of the ripe fruit. This brings back memories of my childhood days, when the false world of supermarkets did not yet lure us or hold the promise of new wonders every day. In those days, food was more valuable than it is today. The work of the farmers received more respect. There was no expiry date on packaging yet, and throwing away edible food was unthinkable.

With the availability of many fruits at any time of the year and the range of ready-made and pre-packaged meals, the relationship to the natural cycle of vegetation is becoming increasingly

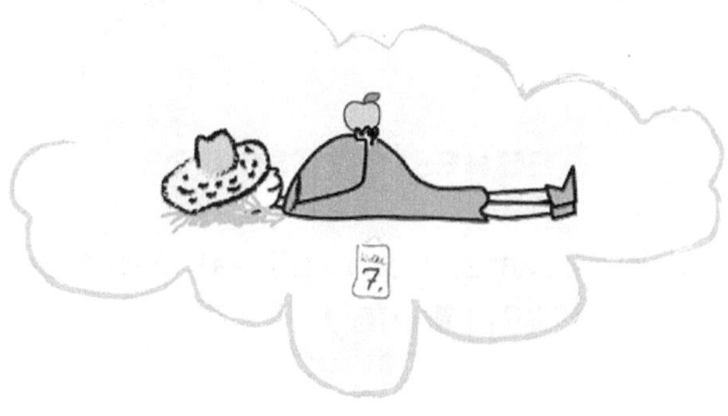

lost. The increasing use of synthetic food additives, such as flavour enhancers, colourings and preservatives, not only changes our taste experiences, but also the physiological value of our food.

I have experienced for myself that only fresh, original ingredients in the diet are the key to good health. It has changed my life for the better, and the intensive preoccupation with it is good for the soul.

This year I have cycled over 3000 kilometres. I'm happy to be able to fulfil all these dreams when I am 50, and I'm happy and grateful that I don't need any medication and have no health problems.

I can often help myself

My relationship with medication has become more cautious since I became healthy. I trust in my self-healing powers and look after my inner balance, which I don't want to disrupt. However, my reservations about medicines remain. I must therefore be careful not to lose complete confidence in them from the outset in case I really need medication.

My intestinal flora now seems to be perfectly in harmony with me and, in return, it stabilises my immune system. My success with it has also been confirmed by the fact that I've not had a cold or skin problems for several years.

My headaches have also decreased as I prevent any tension through regular exercise. But I continue to drink green tea, because my headache is guaranteed to come back when I forget the tea!

Requested recipes

People often ask me what I can still eat. Most people suspect that I now have to follow a very strict diet. But when I explain to them the abundance of food on my table, I'm greeted with a look of disbelief. When I talk about our cooking and baking habits, it draws huge interest. It's then that I realise that, in fact, I cook quite differently and have already learned well how to play by the wholefood rules.

It is actually quite simple: I only use what's ripe in my kitchen. I enjoy a large part of it raw every day. Harvesting and preparing was normal 200 years ago. Asparagus in winter, fresh strawberries from China or cake and bread made from ready-made flour mixture wasn't possible, and I think that was a good thing. Is it really necessary to have everything always available, even if the freshness and taste suffer from it? Have we become too impatient to wait for the natural changing of the seasons?

My friends' curious interest gave me a new idea: I'm a book designer, why don't I write a book about my cooking?

The personal experience that I had with my own health and the right nutrition gave me the self-confidence I needed for this idea. This thought haunted me for the next few weeks. I'll cook my way through all the seasons. I wanted to find the ingredients for this in my garden, in the yard when out picking myself, or in the woods and meadows.

I also saw it as a good exercise for me: it will teach me to be more consistent in my diet.

In addition to these very personal motives, there was also a business aspect: two years ago we won the pitch to be an agency for the marketing concept for German Hiking Day in Fläming in 2012. I'm believe that the book to be a beautiful poster for the region: My region – a health region! I think, with so many reasons, I really have to get started on it!

I like to be inspired by cooking and try something new. But I also love the traditional cuisine of my childhood. So I began to look around in old recipe books in search of something worth preserving, as was once cooked in the time of Queen Luise's. From many suggestions I created a colourful collection, subdivided according to the seasons. The recipes had to meet my "seasonal" criterion and then be fully reinterpreted.

In every season there should be a mixture of soups, baked, boiled and sweet dishes. I therefore took another critical look at my collection and checked which typical products from the

region were not yet represented or were represented too often. It was important to me that all the seasons were given the same coverage, because we always have to eat and at the end of the day, I don't hibernate. But what actually grows in winter?
When I started compiling the recipes, it was autumn. I went through my garden and looked at what was ripe. Besides pumpkins and apples, there were plums, potatoes, red cabbage, savoy cabbage, carrots, turnips, beetroot, courgettes and onions. A friend brought me quinces. On my bike rides I came across elderberries, rose hips and cranberries.

With the start of the one and a half year cooking marathon our cooking habits also changed. The menu was now determined by the season and by our recipes for the cookbook. That was complex, but also very exciting. I prepared many dishes for the first time. The taste experience often surprised us.

Patisson and the Muscat pumpkin had successfully defended their place against the slugs this year. I hollowed out and filled the harvested patissons with a spoon. One Muscat pumpkin was prepared together with the sour rose hip pulp to a creamy soup, another with aromatic apples to a bright orange-red, fruity jam. Since it is slaughtering time in the countryside in autumn, we had potato pancakes with fresh red sausage and sauerkraut. I noticed that you can also bake crispy fritters from sauerkraut. For the savoy cabbage I found an old, simple recipe, the "Fläminger bacon cabbage"; with a little garlic sour cream it tastes very good even without bacon. Also beet pieces in different colours, fried in butter, and caramelized with honey, were sprinkled with fresh parsley and particularly impressed our children. Red cabbage can be more than just a side dish: cream of red cabbage soup with cream topping or a raw vegetable salad made from finely grated red cabbage, black salsify and apples is one of my favourite salads. That's how I cooked my way through the lush, autumn season. It wasn't difficult to find recipes suitable for every fruit, because everything has always had its traditional equivalent in regional cuisine.

Before winter, however, I was worried. What can be harvested in winter? But I quickly realised, there was no need. Many different beets, cabbages and onions and countless preparation options make the winter almost the richest of all the months! So that people didn't have to starve in the cold season in the past, they came up with all kinds of ideas: beets, cabbage and apples were stored for the winter. Fruit, berries and herbs were dried and vegetables pickled. Pickled cucumbers or sauerkraut are a big hit in terms of nutritional physiology and taste and are very popular in Berlin and right as far as the Spreewald. I was fascinated by the variety of uses for onions and sauerkraut: raw vegetable salads, soups, casseroles, lentils, stews and onion or sauerkraut cakes meant that I was completely won over by regional winter cooking.

As a supplement I use wild fruits like medlars, sea buckthorn or rose hips. At the end of the year, Christmas cooking begins with its culinary extras. Roast game, biscuits, poppy-seed cake and fruit bread take care of our "protective shell" against ice and cold: winter bacon.

Medication costs for 2010: 0 Euro.

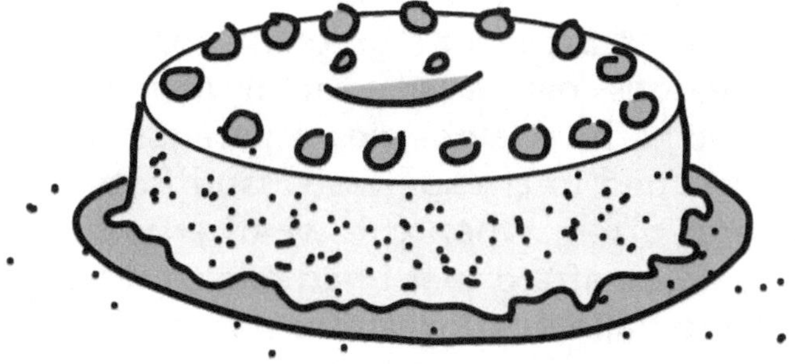

2011

A hobby for the senses

Cooking, photographing and developing recipes has been our only leisure activity for many weeks now. There has been no time to paint and dance. But that's not a bad thing since it's probably just for a transitional period, I thought.

For many people, the most frequently cited reason for not cooking for themselves is a lack of time. I must contradict this, because it is possible to cook tasty and nutritious, simple recipes without spending a lot of time. That's why I prefer simple dishes – good, straightforward cuisine. Because it is these simple dishes, lovingly prepared with good ingredients that inspire. Pan-seared potatoes, vegetable stir-fries with spelt rice, herring with onions and potatoes, curd cheese and linseed oil, potato soup, chicken soup, yeast lentils with plum or apple purée.
For me, cooking means taking time and discovering a slower pace. It makes me happy and trains my senses, a wonderful way to balance everyday life with the computer!

Surprisingly, spring was the biggest challenge. Every day, I looked longingly out of the kitchen window, to see the first thing that peeks out from under the snow. It was the nettles, chickweed and chives. Excellent ingredients for soup, bread and cakes. But the seasons changed at a rapidly increasing pace: salads, radishes, wild herbs, strawberries, asparagus, rhubarb, cherries, and they seemed to change faster and faster. Everything has its time, and often, when the weather was particularly beautiful, I would be afraid that I had missed the best harvest time. If we had to bake or cook dishes two or three times, we would sometimes lose sight of other ingredients that nature offered. As a result, we had to bake and eat the gooseberry cake twice, because the resulting photo did not meet our expectations. This meant that the next planned elder plums had to be postponed. Unfortunately, the elder had almost withered by then! So, in our planning, we always had to pay attention to how quickly nature was set to provide us with its next offering.

Throughout spring, the certainty grew in me that my plan would be successful. For almost nine months I had concentrated almost exclusively on regional products for cooking, frying and baking. We also received a nod of approval from friends and our children, who were repeatedly invited to try our creations. We could not have consumed the bounty from our cookbook production on our own.

Holidays from cooking

Over the summer I planned to go on another bike tour with my friend. This time our journey would take us to the western Baltic Sea. After nine months of regional and seasonal wholefood à la Michaela Barthel, I felt really fit and looked forward to this physical endeavour.
We took the train to Flensburg and planned to arrive in Wismar after six days. We didn't make an exact plan of the day trips or

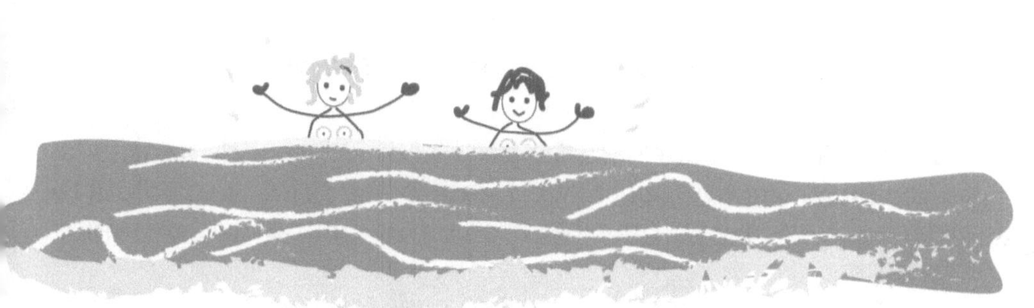

accommodation bookings. We trusted that there would be enough friendly hosts here again. And it was never really a problem to get accommodation for one night. The Baltic Sea between Flensburg and Lübeck is well prepared for spur-of-the-moment cyclists. The advantage is that you can freely choose the length of your tours, depending on your form on the day and the weather. Our stages were different in length. The longest day was 102 kilometres – and we were really happy that day when we had a place to stay overnight – we slept like logs!

The Baltic Sea cycle path mostly runs alongside the sea, but also repeatedly through the very varied hinterland. I enjoy the peace and the wind "between the seas". By bike you can reach secluded places that would be inaccessible by car. We've discovered some nice bathing spots by doing this.

At every port we reached, we refuelled ourselves with a fish sandwich. Even though the roll was made of white flour, this was an "exception" I couldn't avoid since the wholefood fish roll is sadly yet to be invented, and the fresh sea breeze whetted my appetite. We used farm shops and fruit stalls to fill our bags with fresh fruit or vegetables, which we then enjoyed eating at our next break on the beach. The only thing I really missed was my fresh grain breakfast. The breakfast in our holiday accommodation was usually very nice but nevertheless it was very conventional. In the evening we tasted the regional food offered by the guesthouses, with a lavish salad being very important to me. I was fine with all this. I also knew that my risk of intolerance was low thanks to the cycling.

My idea is taking shape

A big folder with countless recipes full of notes and changes lay on my desk. My computer was filled to the brim with colourful pictures. Now it was time for me to think about the design of my book.

A full-page photo should be part of every recipe, because I want to encourage people to cook for themselves. It is important to me not to fool anyone by styling the dish in a way that what you see in the picture is not what you actually eat. The naturalness of the ingredients should also be conveyed through the photography. Taking pictures of the finished dishes was a challenge. My kitchen became a photo studio. My stomach often rumbled loudly between spotlights, steaming pots and aromatic dishes. After the cooking came the plating up, garnishing, lighting and photography. When the pictures were "in the can", the food was cold, but the great thing was there was plenty of variety every day!

In autumn my "year of cooking" was over. We had cooked almost 200 dishes, some of them several times. However, the material was far too extensive in comparison to the planned volume of the book.
To make room, I reduced the baking recipes. Another possible option was to publish a baking book in addition.
So I gave myself more time for editing, and still I felt sure that I could publish the book in time for German Hiking Day 2012.

Medication costs in 2011: 0 Euro.

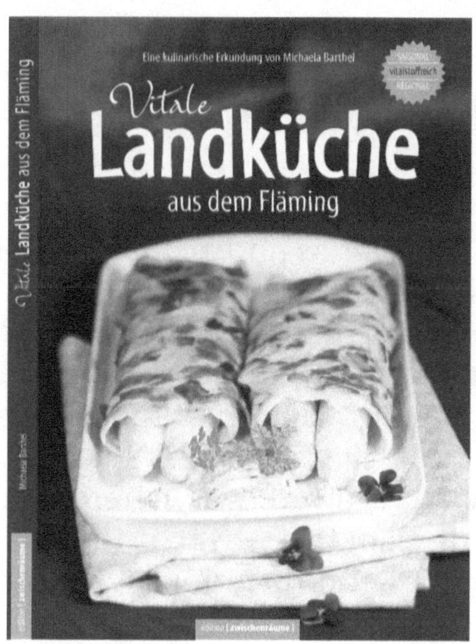

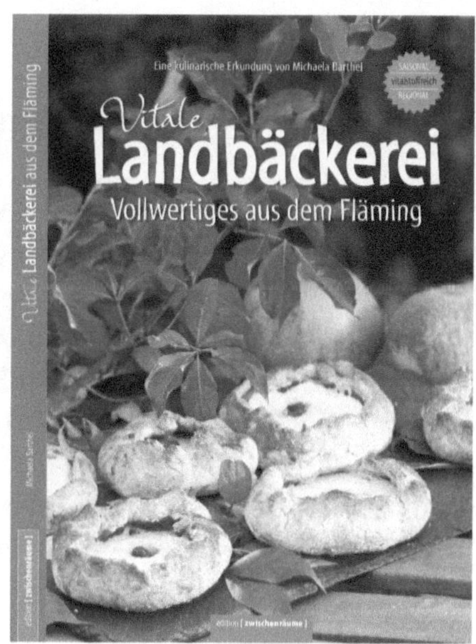

2012

Culinary diversity is growing

I enjoyed leafing through the first chapters of the book. However, some seasons are too abundant and others have too few recipes. There is too much sweet stuff, too few vegetables, too much meat or too little raw food. I want to eat a varied diet in every season of the year, and this should of course be reflected in my book.
At least three days a week, usually late in the evening, the kitchen was busy again. Little by little, the last few gaps were filled. I sent the finished recipes to my friends, who I had long since initiated into my project, for re-cooking and testing. But it wasn't just the filling of these gaps that was a new challenge, so too were the texts and design. All recipes had to be checked again for accuracy of ingredients and measurements. The tips on the recipe pages were also subjected to a critical review.

In June I had achieved it

In June I held my book in my hands: it was published in time for the start of German Hiking Day. My friends and acquaintances, to whom I first showed the book, were enthusiastic and full of praise. For me, this was important confirmation and reward for the effort of the previous weeks and months.
With this momentum behind us, the distribution of the book to bookshops, farm shops and tourist facilities in the region was easy. To my delight, it was very well received everywhere.
The most important lesson I learnt from this was that there is a great interest in how to eat healthy and nutritious local produce all year round.

Basic course

While I was still working on the book, it became increasingly clear to me that I would very much like to complete a basic training course to be a health consultant. Much of what I had worked out in practice I could theoretically consolidate and expand.
 I felt that the Gesellschaft für Gesundheitsberatung (GGB e.V.) would be the right partner for me, because it works independently of economic interests, very much in line with Dr. Bruker. My personal experiences since becoming healthy have given me the push to do this. But I don't want to give up my job and become a health consultant, I want to expand my general education about health and nutrition. The basic course is offered to those with a general interest; there is no obligation to continue.

My sister, who for many years was sceptical about my diet, although she had been suffering from rheumatism for many years, was now also interested in the subject. I had "infected" her and "ignited" her with my book. Catrin agreed on impulse, to my delight, and we decided to attend the course this year instead of doing a bike tour together.

In August, the time had come. We went to Lahnstein. I wanted to use my time on the journey there to visit Waltraut in Kassel. She was not well, the antibody therapy had weakened her body a lot; she could barely walk and suffered from severe pain caused by a poorly sited port. But as always, she was happy and positive and was delighted that we had come. She was filled with joy when she told me that the chemotherapy would soon be over and she had plans to go to rehab again in autumn. She was very optimistic that she would soon be well again.
Waltraut was always particularly happy when she was eating something sweet: "If I'm not allowed whatever I want, but I can have chocolate then I'll treat myself. I won't let that be taken away too"! I gave her these little pleasures from the heart. Today though I know that sugar is the best food for cancer.

The basic training began, and we sweated it out in the literal sense. The lectures on the components of our food and the role of vital substances in nutrition were very theoretical. Saccharides, pyruvic acid, laevulose and galactose were buzzing around in my head looking for a place, because it was the hottest week of summer, and the lecture room in Bruker House has a glass front with a beautiful view to the south. That's also why we had sweat on our forehead when we were learning. This was easier for my sister, because as a PhD biologist, the subject matter was not new territory for her.

Conclusion of the lecture: our food should not be processed or processed as little as possible, nor should it be heated. If it is, it loses its vitality and thus a large part of its vital substances. Vital substances are essential for our health.

On this course, breakfast, lunch and dinner is the animal-protein-free wholefood cuisine: in the morning the fresh grain dish is served and prepared using different methods. Sandwich spreads, rolls and bread also vary daily and taste delicious. The large salad buffet at lunchtimes and in the evenings is very tasty and a nice surprise every day is the warm midday meal. I have been long since been convinced by the intense taste of the nutritious wholefood diet. It is healthy, fresh, natural and the preparation of the food is not difficult. Cooking becomes a symbiosis of fun and health. My concern that an animal-protein-free diet would restrict this experience has been completely unfounded.

The day starts with early morning exercise and breakfast preparation in the training kitchen. This is followed by lectures or group work on various topics: Diet-related diseases of modern society, Construction and function of the locomotor system, Naturopathic treatment, what does our character have to do

with our destiny? Our diet regime, Medical advice from a holistic perspective
and many other topics. The open-minded and cheerful atmosphere in the whole place and among the participants meant that we barely noticed how quickly the week went by.
On our way back, in the car, Catrin raised a completely different subject: "Why don't you write your story? A book that gives others the opportunity to help themselves as well?" "It's so amazing, you're doing so well now. Write it all down." She said. "It could be of use to others too! And you already have experience of writing books!
She's right about what I did to get better, others could do the same. While I was writing my book, I had already thought about this myself, since that would be a much greater help for those affected than my cookbook. But me, write? This is completely different from simply stringing recipes and nice photos together! I couldn't imagine it. It has been so many years. Would I still be able to remember everything?

Fette-Lipide
ungesättigte
Fettsäure

H
$$H-\overset{}{\underset{H}{C}}-\overset{}{\underset{H}{C}}=\overset{}{\underset{H}{C}}-COOH$$

Glutensäure

No, the hurdle seemed too high, especially since I had already decided to publish a baking book next! I had so many ideas in my head and was really looking forward to it! Two books at the same time, I couldn't do that! Nevertheless, a new idea was born, and while I was still prevaricating and trying to get my head around it, she said:
"Do it, you can do it!" I sensed then that the idea was taking hold. But my body fought valiantly against it for a long time.
As soon as my sister arrived home, she bought a grain mill. She also bought two small mills, which her children use regularly to this very day, following her motherly and consistent instruction.
As if that wasn't enough, she also infected her best friend with her pronounced enthusiasm for grain.

Waltraut has gone

In September, completely unexpectedly, I received the news that Waltraut had died. Her husband told me that she went to rehab filled with optimism. She had previously been in hospital for three weeks due to an inflammation of her chemotherapy port. In the last six months, she had been having radiotherapy to her brain because the cancer had metastasised there. The damage to the blood vessels caused by the radiation and the early administration of thrombosis injections had probably led to a fatal reaction. Waltraut died of a brain haemorrhage.
I was really hoping she'd be able to defeat the disease. She was so brave and always optimistic, I admired that about her! Why didn't she get a second chance?

"Look after your body,
so that your soul wants to live in it."
Teresa of Avila

Water, flour and salt are needed for good bread. I love good bread and delicious cake. The smell of fresh bread reminds me of my childhood, of my grandfather's visits to the mill in Neumühle/Elster. Following on from my two uncles, my cousin now continues today to run my grandfather's mill with his son. My grandparents still recognised bread that had been baked honestly, by hand, because they themselves had a bakery in their mill. Cut into thin slices, spread well with butter and salted a little, it was a popular delicacy not only for us children. This experience and the delicious cakes and pies made by my grandmother, my aunt Barbara and my mother have shaped my love of baking and my search for original recipes.
However, I have changed the list of ingredients for my new book a little since I bake with whole foods. I do not use superfine flour, only wholemeal flour. I also want to test the variety of grains to find out which works best in my recipes. I bought oats, rye, spelt, buckwheat and also chickpea flour from the organic shop. I usually grind my grain myself because it con-

tains the most vital substances when freshly ground. The high mineral and fibre content in wholemeal flour is good for your health. Baking requires a little practice because this flour has a different kneading and baking behaviour than superfine flours. I had to practise for quite some time before my breads turned out well, I had to use different kinds of grain, and degrees of grinding as well as play around with the time and temperature factors. The delicious taste was reward enough for that. Wholemeal flours are particularly suitable for savoury baked goods such as bread, vegetable pies, pizzas, pancakes or flat breads. Even fine cakes, pastries and desserts can be made with wholemeal flour without any problems. Combining ground nuts is adds a certain je ne sais quoi.

One reason why I want to write this baking book is for the sweet cakes in particular. Nobody can believe how wonderful cakes and pies taste without sugar! The use of ripe, sweet fruits and regional honey varieties enhances the natural aroma.
I also like to experiment with less common original grain varieties: emmer, einkorn, barley or millet. Much from the past is at risk of being forgotten; I'm pleased to have discovered these things in old cookbooks and bake them according to my current nutritional experiences.
Baking takes time. It's about doing something good for yourself and getting involved at a pace set by nature: in this case, the pace of countless hard-working bacteria and yeasts. The more time a dough has to rise, the finer the taste. I like this relaxed manner.

In September, my mother celebrates her 80th birthday. When I asked her what she wanted for this new year in her life, she responded with, "You know what I'd like, Micha? I'd like a grain mill." My parents now also want to prepare a fresh grain dish every day. That's such a gift for me, too.

Farewell Snoopy

The way to the office had become too far for our dog, Snoopy. He was 12 years old. He wanted to run, but only managed shorter distances. In March, his condition continued to deteriorate, he buckled when walking on his front paws. Now he could hardly leave the house. I became painfully aware that the nutrition for animals is also not appropriate for the species. He mostly ate dry muesli food, always sugar-free, we made sure of that. We also fed him tinned food. Neither of which is species-appropriate. Now we gave him a large portion of fresh grain with cream, grated apple or finely grated carrots every day, because he loved it so much.

We could no longer hope for an improvement. The vet suspected spondylosis as the cause of his restrictions in movement. But the x-ray revealed more: The tumour was back and it was the same size as it was before. And when he buckled again, his neck and right front paw were stiff.

I held him in my arms when he was euthanised. And I knew he'd gone forever. He was there for the children when we had far too little time for them and he was there for me when I was sick. He cheered me up and made me laugh on so many occasions! And when I stroked him, it was always my soul that soared.

I'm grateful to him for the time he spent with us. I never thought we would all miss those lovely brown eyes and the golden wagging tail!

I'm often asked: "Will you get a new dog?" I don't think about that. He has a permanent place in my heart after all these years. I can well imagine that he will never disappear from it and I'm comfortable with that thought. I promised him I'd walk our big circuit every day, for at least an hour.

Medication costs in 2012: 0 Euro.

2013

The topic is fun

Since the publication of my book "Vitale Landküche" [Nutritious Country Cooking] I have received a lot of response, from the press. In February I was invited to the MDR television programme "Hauptsache Gesund" [Focus on Health]. The basic theme of my book was in line with the focus of the programme: chronic inflammatory intestinal diseases. I had the opportunity to talk about my illness and how I managed to find a way out of this nightmare. My book "Vitale Landküche" became known nationwide and, by the end of April, the book was out of print; this success blew me away! After the television report I received numerous calls, e-mails and very personal letters from those affected, who were also desperately looking for a way out of the disease. These many personal stories were a decisive incentive for me to drive forward the work on this book, "Farewell Colitis".

But what sort of book was it meant to be? I wanted to write a book that I wished I could have read when I had almost given up hope myself. I then started to meticulously compile and sort through all documents, experiences and stories, so I could arrange them into a timeline. How long would it take? I guess a few months. After a while, I realised that this would mean once again facing the unpleasant sides of the disease. I realised that I had to write about very personal things and about facts I've never shared with anyone before. Was I going to be okay?
The project quickly became more extensive. I had to check memories and events for their relevance to the disease or to the development of the disease. Many things only became clear to me when I was writing, and every time I thought I was almost finished, new memories would come to the fore, a new insight

would come to mind or the connection would become clearer. I also felt that there were many things that I couldn't write about because I couldn't even explain them myself. How could I tell others what I didn't understand myself? With whom could I exchange information? Of course I could talk to Helmut about anything, but I also needed someone who didn't know anything about my life, who could help me with all the technical issues. For this reason, I decided to take the advanced training course for health consultants after all. I needed more experience on the causes of illness, and I was looking for answers about myself. So I registered for the course in August.

It occurred to me that I still get a headache if I don't drink my green tea early! There's no green tea in Lahnstein! I'm going to try now to wean myself off it. Could I be free of my addiction before I go on the course?

Life without green tea

From conversations in Lahnstein I knew how to solve the problem. I wanted to try this out myself before the course. Since I only drink loose tea, it's straightforward. I've reduced the amount of

"green leaves" in my tea strainer every day. The taste decreased and so did the colour. I didn't feel a headache at all. After two weeks, all I drank in the morning was clear water. I didn't get a single headache.

I now only drink a cup of green tea on special occasions. The headaches didn't come back either. I was amazed how easy it was! Why hadn't I tried this before? For decades I thought I could only avoid headaches by drinking coffee or tea. You really just have to start! It was also helpful for me that I had learned how to relax properly.

From organic to abdominal brain

In August I went on the advanced training course at the Bruker house in Lahnstein. During this course I wanted to gain clarity on many questions that came to me when writing my book. So I wanted to find more answers to the question on why I got ulcerative colitis in the first place. The answer that it was an autoimmune disease was not enough for me.

The range of events this week was very extensive. The determining topics were lifestyle-related illnesses, basic knowledge about our nervous system and about cardiovascular diseases. Further group work on disease-causing diets and on nutrition research findings regarding animal protein-free foods. Although it has been scientifically proven for over 50 years that vegetable proteins also contain all essential amino acids, it is still commonly taught in conventional nutrition that this is not the case. Furthermore, the misconception that a healthy diet is accompanied by a high protein content was dispelled. That was informative because preparing food without milk, cheese, quark and eggs is still new territory for me. Since everything that's prepared here tastes excellent to me, I would like to pursue the topic further.

We also received extensive information on the topics of organic farming, organic food, organic seals and genetic engineering. Given the large number of seals of origin and quality on organic products, it is often difficult to find your bearings and make the right decisions.

A new Kneipp facility has been built in the Bruker garden, which we use daily after morning exercise and during breaks. Cold water applications: this is something that fills me with enthusiasm because I always feel really well afterwards. So I had an idea, once I was back in my garden, I would find suitable solutions, that wouldn't be too much trouble. Of course, the simplest thing is a daily early morning walk.

What insights this week will help me with my book? There's a lot I still have to think about: according to Dr. Bruker, diseases are divided into three groups: Diet-related, lifestyle-related and diseases caused by environmental pollution. I had found out for myself that my illness obviously had something to do with my diet. But what influence did my lifestyle have on the disease? Lifestyle-related diseases can only be understood if you consider the living human being as a whole. So even those things that have been completely messed up in our lives have influenced us, because illness comes from insult, I learn. Living together in the family, relationships between children, with teachers, colleagues or neighbours and many more, can be a role-playing game. I realise that this is also the box I'm in right now, in relation to my book, sitting and rummaging around in it, like in an old family photo album.

But how can the stresses of life make a person organically ill? What is the mechanism behind it? There is a link, I learnt, between the human being as a unity of body and soul and his environment. The linking system is the nervous system, especially the vegetative system. We not only have a brain in our head, but also a so-called abdominal brain. Eighty percent of the nerve fibres that run between the two systems lead from the abdomen to the brain and only twenty percent in the opposite direction. As a result, the abdominal brain reacts extremely sensitively and often much more intensively. Psychological and abdominal stress factors, such as stress at work or in the family and poor nutrition, can lead to disorders. Surely everyone at some point has had an upset stomach or a gall bladder twinge. These popular expressions describe the temporary physical reaction to a negative emotional state or stress. If these stresses persist for a long time, they lead to serious illnesses. I had long suspected that permanent occupational stress and excessive demands during my periods of illness were certainly a cause of any new flare-ups. Perhaps they were even more important to me than nutrition. I don't feel stable enough just because of the change in diet. This was confirmed in the lectures that Dr. Mathias Jung gave us on the topics "My Character – My Fate" and "Depression – the exhausted soul". These were important topics that helped me to better understand myself and my actions. There was a lot to process. My folder of this week's personal notes was very extensive. Now I've gathered a lot of material for my book, the work can continue.

The days here usually ended very late as we still went on very long walks following the exhausting courses. When I was in my room and also during the long train ride, which was made even longer due to the spring floods, I wrote this/my story in great detail.

Practical experience

I wanted to use and try out what I had learned. Once I was back home, I grabbed a suitable winter bucket. Thanks to the rainwater in my tool shed, this was always freshly filled. As a crowning conclusion to my early morning walk, I now have what's called: Get in the bucket! Autumn came and it became a little cooler, but I felt that I could actually always stay outside longer. Especially since I didn't suffer from cold feet at all anymore! This morning session refreshes me, perks me up and somehow I've become addicted to it!

For arm showers, I use the water butt. It does not take much effort to ladle both arms evenly with the fresh cold water, then I brush off the water and wait for my arms to warm up by themselves. I deliberately seek simple helpful ways; if it is too complicated or too costly, I can't keep up with it.

Since I started to change my diet to whole foods twelve years ago, dental problems have become a thing of the past. In particular, giving up food containing refined sugar has played a decisive role here. When brushing my teeth, I now use a mild organic herbal toothpaste which does not contain fluorine. A small amount is sufficient because it does not have to foam up. I'm very careful not to swallow any of it! Because everything I swallow arrives in my intestine at some point!

I now only wash my hair every seven to ten days. My scalp is used to it, and oil production is regulated. I also brush my hair "the wrong way" daily, with a natural bristle brush. This invigorates my head early on and the hair becomes relaxed and almost arranges itself. I haven't used body lotion for a long time. I want my skin to be able to care for itself. Alongside cold water applications, that is the best form of skin protection. I'm very happy with my skin now, it's smooth and feels great.

In very cold weather, a fingertip of sunflower oil on my lips helps. When the skin looks tired, I make a quark honey oil pack or a face peel with healing clay. I mix a level teaspoon of healing clay with a little sunflower oil or linseed oil, and rub it into my face and décolleté. The oil ensures that the healing clay adheres well. After twenty minutes I wash everything off, my skin is refreshed and can breathe better again and feels soft. A fine face brush is also really pleasant to use. I no longer have conjunctivitis, dry eyes or skin irritations. This is also tells me that my immune system is doing well right now. I now have bad reactions now with liquid toilet block. After putting it in the toilet bowl, the next day I have noticed skin eczema. It was only after a few days that I associated the problem with the cleanser, which obviously emits vapours. After removing the container from the toilet, the eczema disappeared within just one day.

Healing clay helps me with light joint pain (as a drink). Every day I drink 3 teaspoons of healing clay, one hour before each meal, dissolved in half a glass of water. I have found that the pain then decreases or even disappears completely. A layer of boiled and crushed floury potatoes, wrapped in a rectangular linen cloth, works wonders for joint pain.

Nutritious Country Bakery –

Nutritious food from Fläming is the title of my new book. The choice to have an autumnal theme on the cover was well suited to the current season. For this book, too, I spent a year "baking" my way through the products of the region. I'm thrilled with the wholefood baking, it's good for me. Over 70 recipe suggestions show what is possible with wholemeal flour. Next to the

classics of bread and rolls, there are vegetable pies and filled omelettes for warm, wholesome lunches. When developing my recipes, I was surprised to discover that almost all vegetables can be used in cakes or tarts – whether beetroot, pumpkin or sauerkraut!
Of course, the book also contains a variety of sweet treats. Sugar is strictly replaced with honey or ripe fruits.

Why am I not a vegetarian?

Vegetarian nutrition is primarily an ethical issue. Besides vegetable-based foods, vegetarians only eat products derived from living animals, such as milk, eggs and honey. They avoid meat and fish and products made from them, such as sausage, gelatine or lard. I can completely understand this thinking.
However, not killing animals does not automatically lead to a healthy diet. Sugar, extract flours, industrially processed vegetable fats and convenience foods made from them are consumed without limitation by vegetarians. They also consume food supplements such as artificial vitamins, colourings, flavours and preservatives. Substitute products, such as vegan salami, tofu sausage, soy products or margarine are designed foods that have long since lost their connection to nature.
I don't find it difficult to do without meat, sausage and milk. Now and then I'll have fish and goat's or sheep's cheese – I wouldn't want to live without these things just yet. But I love to stick my finger in thick cream or try fresh, cold country butter with home-made bread. Butter and cream are as important to me as chocolate used to be. My diet should be suitable for me, I want to feel well on it. What counts is good taste, and my appetite can decide what my body needs.

Medication costs in 2013: 0 Euro

2014

Lecture with taste

The past few months have shown me that interest in proper nutrition is huge. The reasons are very diverse. As such, my event – a combination of a lecture explaining whole foods in detail and a tasting buffet was very rewarding. After the theory there is always practice, the participants were then able to enjoy the wholefood experience on site. The event is entitled: "How I became healthy by changing what I eat". I am invited by bookshops, associations and self-help groups. The great response is a resounding success for me, especially as I get to see how enthusiastic and motivated the attendees are when they say goodbye to me personally.

The idea for the series of events came about as a result of my books: how do I answer the many questions, e-mails and calls that I keep getting? I'm now able to answer them at my events. Part of the practical session is a demonstration with my grain mill and those interested can join in. With these events, my aim is to encourage others to find ways out of their illness. I enjoy working with people who feel responsible for their own health and who tell me about their successes.

On these days the computer stays switched off. In the publishing house, the smells are tempting because we are baking and cooking all day long!

We have been baking our own daily bread for about two years – a heavy sourdough tin loaf with 80 percent rye and some spelt and a tang that you can still easily taste on the tongue after baking – that is our classic! We serve it with cold butter with herbs or home-made plum jam. Baking bread is meditation. To knead a dough, to work it lovingly and gently and to give it the time and warmth it needs, trains my senses and caresses my soul.

To gain tips from an experienced practitioner and exchange experiences, I've already participated twice in a weekend baking seminar with the master baker and health consultant, Ute Olk. A wholemeal baking seminar with the Plötzblog baker also gave me a lot of practical experience. Here I was able to deepen my knowledge of grains and flours as well as dough management. Baking together with like-minded people was a pleasure and was rewarded with a variety of successful breads, cakes, rolls, pastries and casseroles. The icing on the cake was an almost 30-year-old batch of sourdough that we received at the end of Ute Olk's course.

And now, dear readers, thank you for accompanying me through so many years, I've finished this book now and I've got a good feeling that it tells you all the important stuff. Meanwhile I have lots of new ideas flying around in my head. But on some days, there an internal struggle going on and raging desire inside me: I want to start painting again, to put my feelings and ideas on canvas and let the colours take effect.
That's what I'm going to do next.

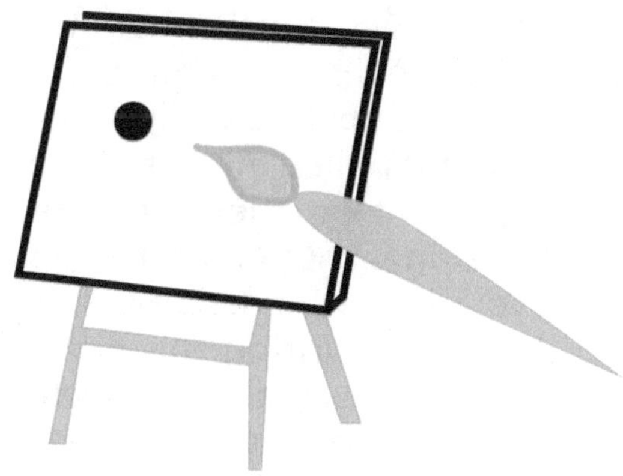

Epilogue 2019

It has been 23 years since the horrid disease took possession of my body and it wouldn't leave for a long time. For seven long years I had to fight to get rid of it. It wasn't until I realised that changing my diet was the key to healing. I only conquered the disease when I had consistently nourished myself with a nutritious wholefood diet and had found my own life rhythm. Today, I am well. I managed to get everything back that I thought I had lost forever and irretrievably. An autonomous life, my wonderful family, my work and my future.

In my quest to cure colitis, I would have wished for more than just medication right from the start. Unfortunately, the health system has repeatedly put the brakes on alternative approaches. Only chance has put me on the right track.

Maybe today it's a lot easier for those affected to get information from the Internet about alternative treatments. There is also a broader public debate on the impact of nutrition on our health.

E-mails, letters, phone calls and many conversations at my events show me, however, that people affected by autoimmune diseases still know too little about the connection between nutrition and their disease. Changing our diets to a nutritious wholefood one is obviously still underestimated as an important treatment. But it pulled me out of the deepest nightmare of my life. An important experience for me was the book "Darm mit Charm" [Intestines with Charm]. Many things that I experienced and discovered, which I describe in this book, I was able to understand through writing this book. It confirmed my experiences! It's so easy, why didn't a doctor explain it to me?

Today I can leave the house whenever I want. I can go to work without fear and worry. I feel healthy and safe, and I enjoy the good feeling in my body, my healthy skin, my thick hair and my strength. I enjoy spoiling myself and my family with good, homemade dishes every day. The rheumatism has also completely disappeared in the last three years. Everything takes time.

For the participants at my events I am often the living proof of a possible way out of this illness. This holds lot of responsibility for me. Since it is not always possible for me to answer the many questions and requests for help, there is now a Part Two entitled "Go with your Gut Instinct" – 13 stories from others who have successfully made the journey out of the condition. I have also published a Guide to Wholefoods for all the family, in which I answer many of the questions I have been asked over the last 5 years about changing my diet to wholefoods. This includes 220 simple recipes for everyone.
And if you want to, write down your story, if you have defeated the disease. Send me your very personal experiences, setbacks, consequences... honestly and authentically, so even more sufferers can be encouraged and help can be given.

Now you are holding in your hands the revised 2nd edition as an ebook. I wish you to find your way out of the illness, back to a life that you wish for. It is important to believe in yourself, believe in your body's self-healing powers and stay consistent.
I wish you all the best and, above all, I wish you good health.
Yours Michaela Barthel

Since you can only find out about this book on the Internet, I would be grateful if you tell others about it or write a review – so that other people may also find help.

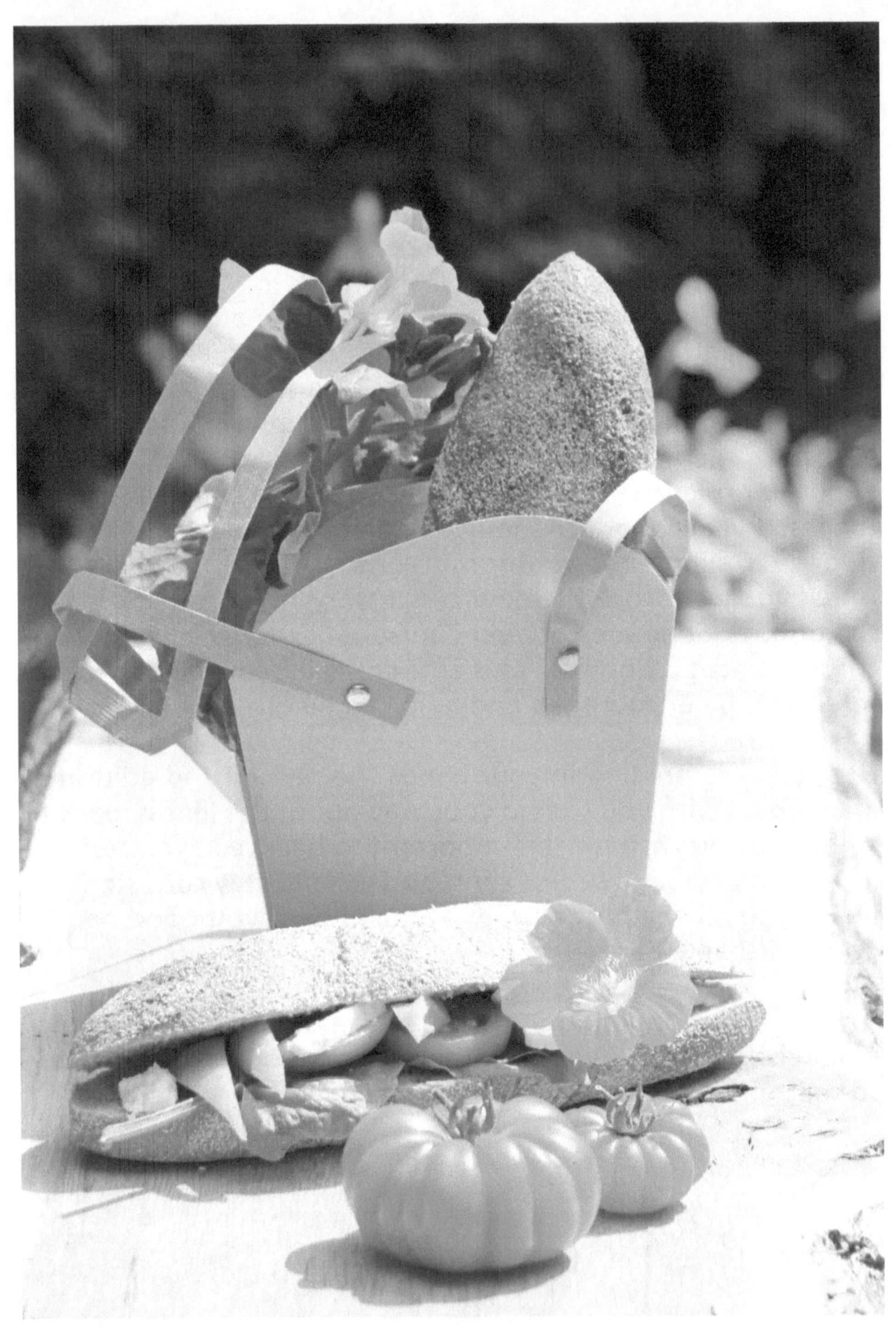

Baking with whole grain

Whole foods

What does "wholesome" and "rich in vital substances" mean?

If the food is natural, it contains all the substances our organism needs to stay healthy in the long term. In addition to the basic nutrients, these include the large group of vital substances: proteins, carbohydrates and fats.

What makes up these vital substances? Fat-soluble and water-soluble vitamins, minerals, trace elements, enzymes, fatty acids in natural compounds, fragrances and flavourings and fibres, also called dietary fibres. These are sufficiently present in natural foods, because the less processed a food is, the more vital substances are still contained within it. The vital substances ensure a functioning metabolism and thus promote an intact immune system. Diet-related diseases hardly stand a chance.

What is so wrong with our modern diet?

In the days of our great-grandparents, many foods came straight from the field or market onto the table. There was only that which was available seasonally and regionally or which was naturally preserved. Fresh food contained all the vital substances we needed for a healthy life. The bread of the poor was brown bread, the wholemeal bread. With increasing industrialisation and the fight against hunger, processing of food began. The aim was to ensure that food was always available, could be stored for a long time and financially affordable. In this way, foods rich in vital substances became foods low in vital substances.

Decades of malnutrition
can lead to which diseases?

1.   Dental decay, dental caries, periodontosis and malocclusions. The latter as a consequence of the poor nutrition of previous generations.

2.   Diseases of the musculoskeletal system, rheumatic diseases (arthrosis, arthritis, damage to the spine and intervertebral discs).

3.   All metabolic diseases, such as obesity, diabetes, liver damage, gallstones, kidney stones, gout.

4.   Most diseases of the digestive organs as well as constipation, liver, gallbladder, pancreas, small and large intestine diseases, digestive and fermentation disorders.

5.   Vascular diseases, for example arteriosclerosis, heart attack, stroke and thrombosis.

6.   Lack of defence against infection, which is manifested in recurrent catarrhs and inflammations of the respiratory tract, so-called colds, and inflammations of the renal pelvis and bladder.

7.   Most allergies.

8.   Some organic diseases of the nervous system.

9.   Malnutrition also plays a significant role in the development of cancer.

What belongs on the whole food table?

1.   Grain capable of germination to meet the need for vitamin B1 and other vital substances. Like no other food, it contains almost all the important minerals such as iron, magnesium, calcium, water and fat-soluble vitamins and enzymes. Since these

ingredients are mostly found in raw, freshly ground grain, the daily fresh grain dish is of great importance in wholemeal cuisine.

2.   Grain is also served in heated form, as cereal porridge and soup, wholemeal bread, wholemeal noodles, unpeeled rice and other wholemeal products.

3.   Fresh food: As an important supplier of valuable vital substances, fresh fruit and vegetables, also prepared as salads or vegetable platters, are a guaranteed provider of the most varied vital substances.

4.   Natural fats such as butter, cream, nuts and almonds, seeds such as sesame, linseed, linseed cake, pumpkin seeds or sunflower seeds, as well as cold-pressed vegetable oils from first pressing.

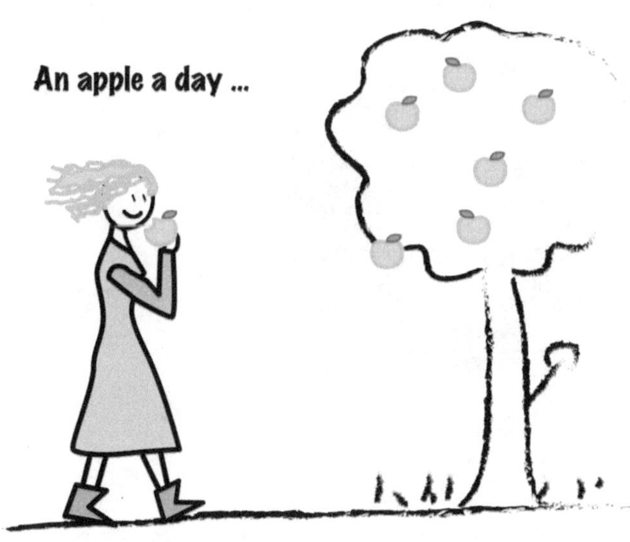

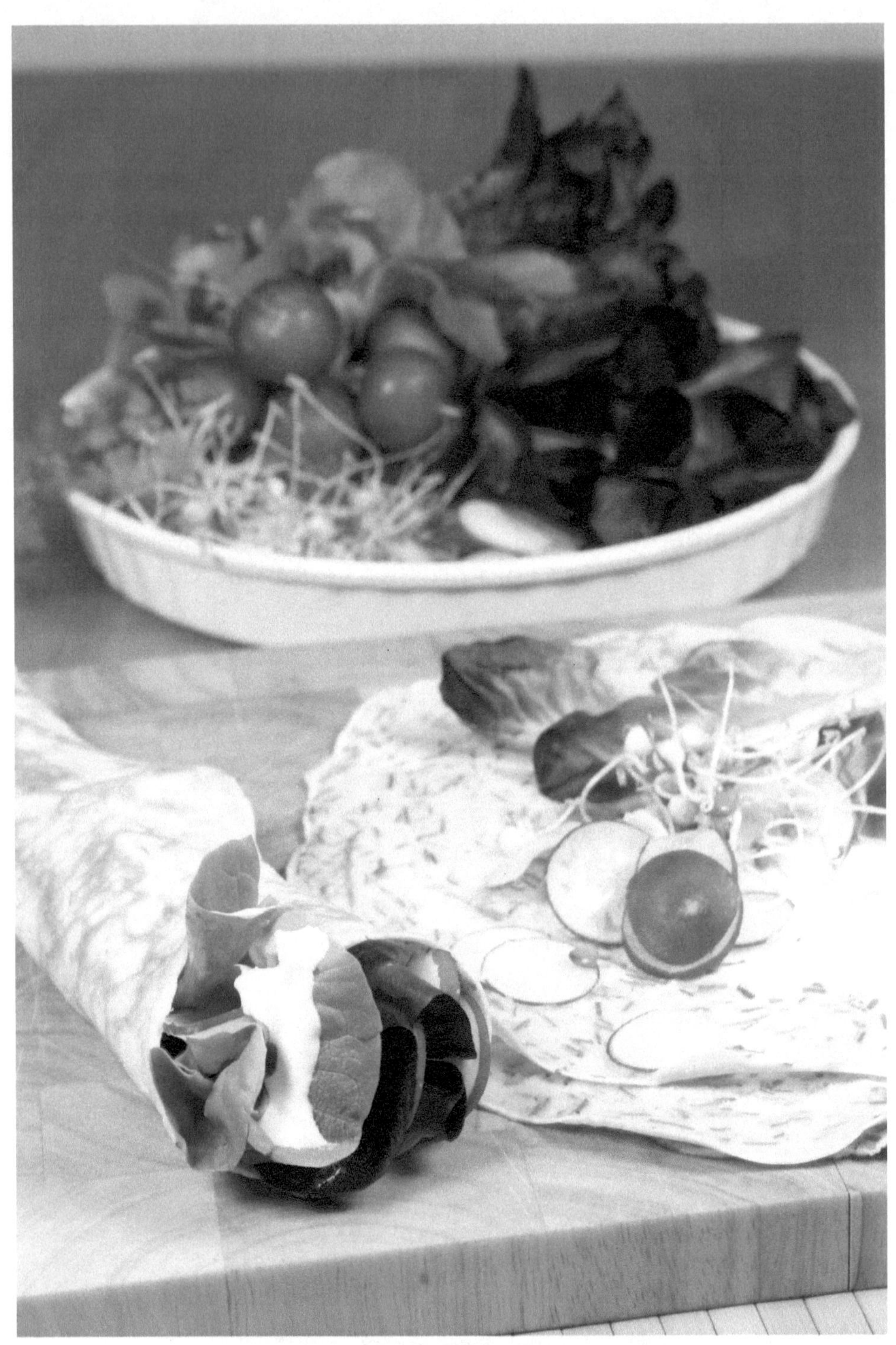

Corn flat bread with spring vegetables

What should you absolutely avoid?

1. All types of refined sugars such as: white sugar, brown sugar, fructose, dextrose, lactose, malt sugar, whole cane sugar, sucanate, original sweetness, original sugar, Ra padura, syrup, apple syrup, pear syrup, maple syrup, agave syrup, molasses, frutilose, barley malt, maltodextrin and many more – as well as all foods sweetened with these.

2. Superfine flours / type flours and all foodstuffs made from them. These are all flour products that are not made from whole grains.

3. Processed fats like: margarine, ordinary frying fats, refined oils and all foods containing them.

4. Juices, cooked fruit, dried fruit, and this is especially true for people with liver, gall bladder, stomach and intestinal sensitivities.

Eat ...

1. always raw vegetables first; and plenty of them.

2. three real, wholesome meals a day.

3. what your body is whispering to you to eat, sharpen your senses when shopping.

4. in peace and quiet and enjoy it. Don't just refuel!

5. together. Don't forget to decorate the table.

6. Colourful foods, because the eyes eat with you.

7. food from the region, from the garden, from the market or game from forests and fields.

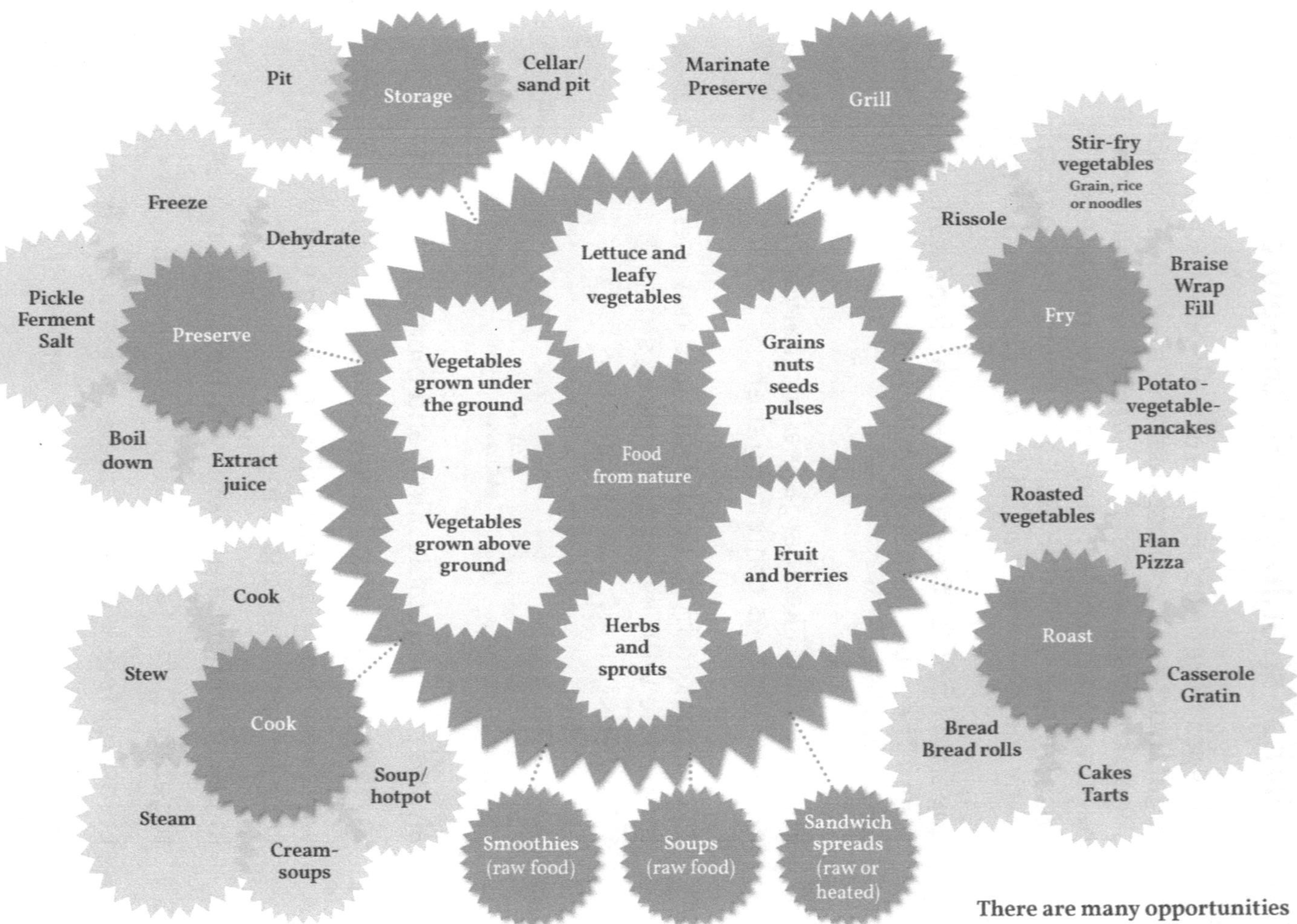

There are many opportunities

My cooking ideas graphic

There were often days when I had no idea what to cook. I would come home from work, my head was empty, I felt exhausted. I looked into the vegetable fridge in the cellar, in my crates and the garden, and I could only think of what I had prepared before, but I didn't feel like doing it! For days like these, I developed my cooking ideas graphic:

In the middle are the basic products of wholefood cuisine, i.e. grain, seeds, vegetables and fruit, berries, salad, nuts and herbs. Starting from the middle, all the processing options are displayed. I can now choose a method of preparation of my choice for what I have just bought.

This is what celery looks like, for example:
I can grate celery raw and make a celery-pear salad with nuts, cut into slices, roast or grill like schnitzel, serve a celery sauce with baked beetroot, cook celery soup, make a celery-potato mash, prepare as sweet-sour celery or as celery-potato-apple gratin and much more.

And for beetroot: I can grate beetroot raw and make a beetroot-apple salad with nuts or a beetroot-sauerkraut salad with cream. Beetroot tart, beetroot-pumpkin cake, baked beetroot, like baked potatoes, or cream of beetroot soup is just as delicious as a ratatouille with beetroot and winter vegetables, a colourful vegetable stir-fry or fried beetroot with mashed potatoes. If you like, you can also marinate them or cook them as a vegetable garnish and serve them with herbal sour cream.
www.vitale-landkueche.de

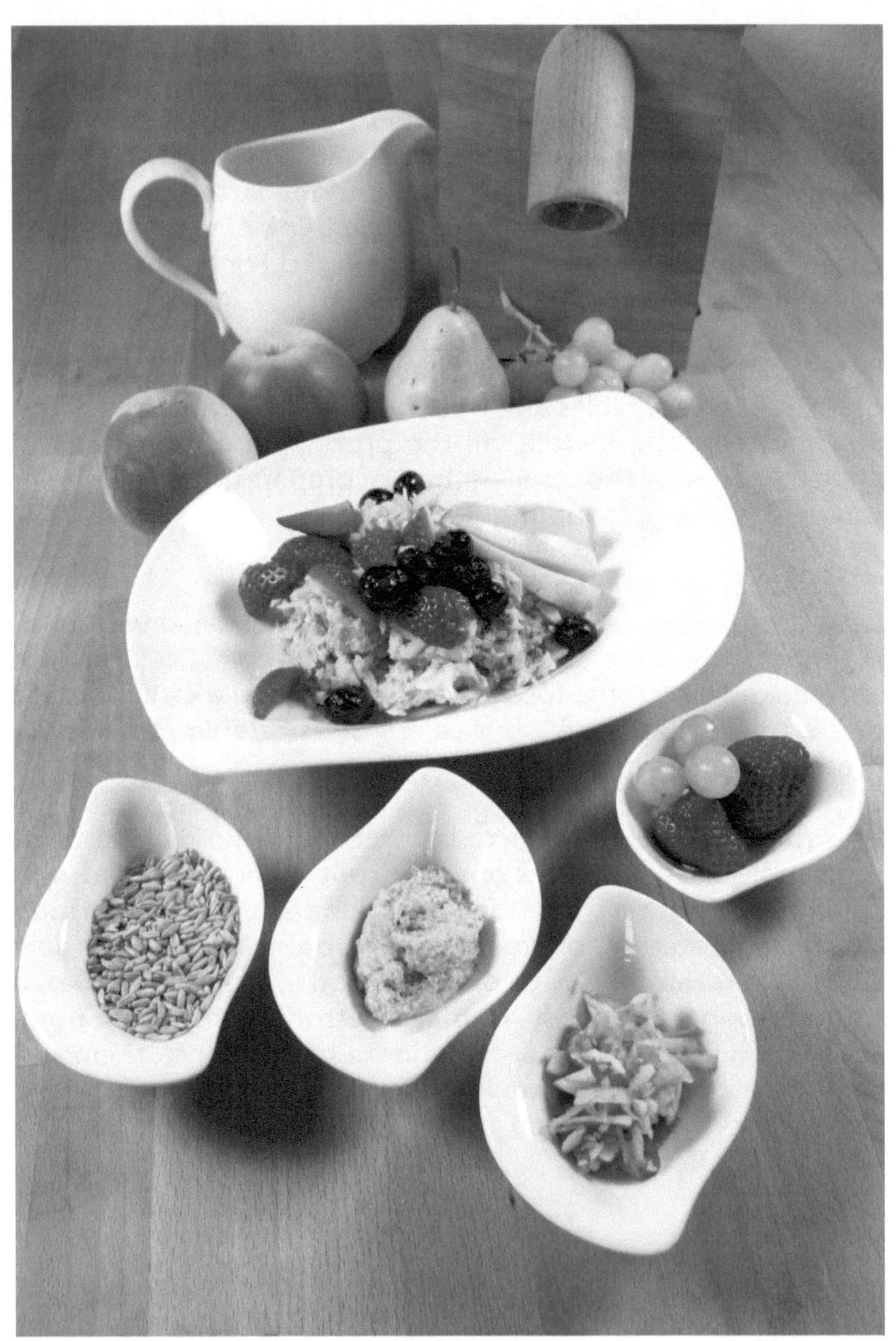

The fresh grain breakfast

Simple basic recipes for beginners
or for inspiration

1.
Grain-fruit-fresh food
The fresh grain dish according to
Dr. Max-Otto Bruker:

Preparation time: max. 10 minutes.

Utensils:
Grain grinder (an old coffee grinder or blender is also suitable), sharp knife, 10 to 15 cm long, large wooden board, grater, large bowl, salad spoon.

Preparation (for 2 persons):
100 g (6 heaped tbsp = 100 g) freshly ground spelt, rye, wheat or any other cereal. Mix the flour with unboiled tap water to a porridge and leave at room temperature for several hours (even overnight). Soaking the grain makes it easier for the body to digest.
The next day: 1 tsp lemon juice for the freshness, 2 grated apples to make the porridge airy, 1 cut banana to make the porridge creamy. 40 g hazelnut, walnut or sunflower seeds make it crunchy and other, preferably seasonal fruits.
2 tbsp organic whipped cream, refine the taste, and with fresh (or in winter frozen) berries to garnish, you'll have the perfect finish.

Some hints for fresh grain dishes:

1. Oats, barley, rye, millet, emmer, einkorn, kamut or buckwheat can also be used as grains. Do not soak oats and buckwheat!
2. The preparation according to Dr. Evers recommends the use of germinated grains. One type of grain is rinsed with

cold tap water in a flat sieve or germination tray, covered with a cloth, for example, and placed on the window sill. This process is repeated twice a day. The grain must be germinated by variety, as the germination period is different for each. After 2 to 4 days 1 to 3 mm long sprouts appear. Then the grain is nutty and soft and can be used for the fresh grain dish.

3. Grain can also be crushed, i.e. flaked.
4. During berry season you can stock up with fresh berries, for example during the self-picking season, the berries are frozen in small portions for the winter.
5. The cream can also be added to the fresh grain without being whipped, but shaken up, which saves some time.
6. If you want a larger portion of fresh grain, simply add more fruit: Pear, plum, peach, apricot; and in winter pineapple, oranges, kiwi.
7. Linseed cake (residue from the oil production), ground lin seed, sunflower seeds, almonds or coconut pieces spice up the whole thing.
8. The fresh grain dish can be enjoyed early or as lunch – then it is soaked in the morning, and the fruit can be added fresh in the office.

2. Fresh food salads
made from vegetables and fruit

Preparing a raw food platter or a salad takes no longer than 10 minutes and can even result in a sufficient meal on its own.
Raw food is easy to prepare, anyone can do it! You need: 1 large board, 1 knife, 1 grater, 1 large bowl, 1 large spoon and a screw-top jar with whisk for the dressing.

Vegetables are brushed until they are clean and free of soil. Bad or soft spots are generously removed. If possible, do not peel the vegetables! Only if the skin is woody or fibrous is it removed, as a large part of the important vital substances are located under the skin. Some vegetables can also be blanched briefly and then peeled (e.g. beetroot). Almost every vegetable can be eaten raw. Exceptions are: Potatoes, beans and some mushrooms.

One third to half of each meal should be fresh food. The fresh food is ALWAYS consumed before the warm meal. This means that the supply of vital substances is ideal if you use a vegetable variety grown above and below ground and combine it with fresh fruit and leaf salad.
Regional, ripe vegetables and fruit are preferable. It should also be organically grown. Foods that ripen at the same time usually go well together in terms of taste. Salads change with the seasons. I also pay attention to an appetising colour combination when selecting the ingredients.

In winter, I recommend a warm-cold salad. Then my salad is often the starter and main course in one. I eat one part of the vegetables steamed, grilled or braised, e.g. braised cabbage, braised cucumbers, grilled peppers, steamed mushrooms, fried potatoes, and the larger part raw. The warm vegetables are arranged in the middle of the plate, the raw vegetables or the salad around it. Not to forget in winter: Some pickled vegetables or sauerkraut. Then there is no hot meal afterwards. Serve with a dressing, a cold salsa verde or simply sour cream with herbs and garlic. Grain, rice, millet, amaranth or wholemeal pasta, cooked in vegetable stock, are also the perfect warm complement.
Herbs, colourful flowers, especially in spring, and wild fruits in autumn enrich my salads.

For my salads I have a "rotating system". Every day I replace one variety of three vegetables with something new. That's why there's a different salad every day. There are, for example: Red cabbage- black salsify-apple salad or red cabbage-Jerusalem artichoke-apple salad, broccoli-Jerusalem artichoke-apple salad. Due to the variety of vegetables there are countless possible combinations! You have to find out for yourself what tastes best to you.

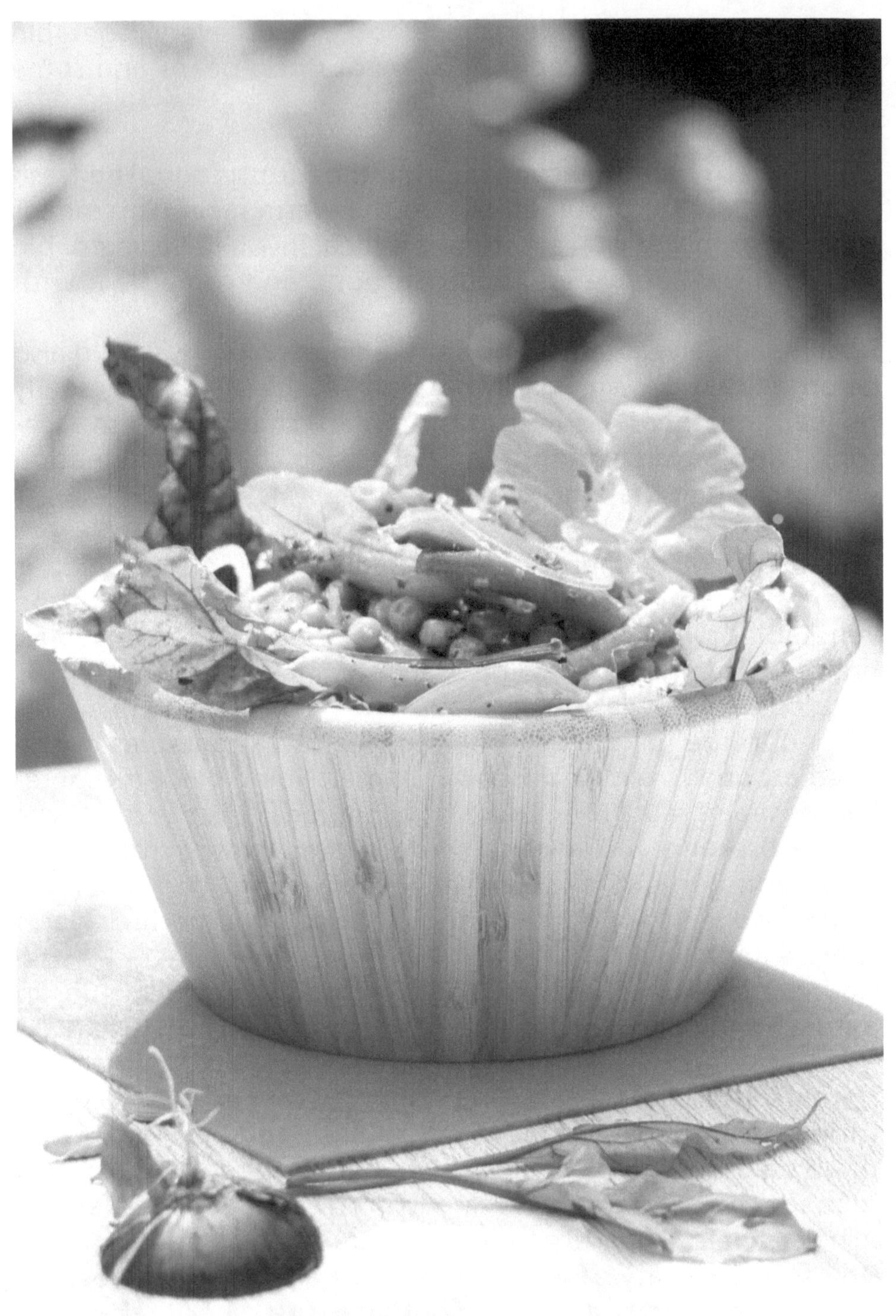

Fresh salad: Walking through the garden ...

Salad 1:
Carrot – Kohlrabi – Apple

Grate carrot, kohlrabi and apples in equal parts and mix with roasted sunflower seeds. Arrange on a plate with red lettuce and dressing.

Salad 2:
Carrot – Courgette – Apple

Grate carrot, courgette and apples in equal parts and mix well with roasted sunflower seeds. Arrange on a plate with red and green lettuce and dressing.

My favourite salad: Salad 3:
Red cabbage – black salsify – apple

Grate red cabbage, black salsify (unpeeled) and apples in equal parts and mix well with chopped nuts and white dressing. The salad is served on a plate with lamb's lettuce.

Salad 4:
Chicory or Chinese cabbage – Orange – Apple

Finely chop the cabbage, peel the orange and cut into small pieces, grate the apples and mix well with roasted sunflower seeds and finely chopped candied orange peel. Arrange on a plate with baby spinach or salad.

Salad 5:
Celery – carrots – pear or apple

Grate celery, carrot and apples in equal parts and mix well with chopped walnuts. Season to taste with lemon juice and cream, decorate with lamb's lettuce.

Salad 6:
Mushrooms – red beet – baby spinach – apple or banana

Slice and sauté the mushrooms, grate the beetroot, cut the apples or pears into fine pieces and mix with chopped walnuts and arrange on the spinach. Add: Potato vinaigrette or simply oil and vinegar.

Salad 7:
Broccoli – red pepper – apple – walnuts

Coarsely grate the broccoli and apple, cut the peppers into very fine pieces and mix with chopped walnuts and white dressing.

Salad 8:
Fennel – apple – orange

Roughly grate the fennel, cut the apples and oranges into small pieces, add 4 tbsp sunflower seeds and mix everything. Serve with lamb's lettuce and dressing.

3.
Dressings for salads

For a variety of flavours: juice of an orange, tomato paste, the purée of wild fruits, such as rose hip, sea buckthorn, sloe, chokeberry, rowanberry or sugar-free, homemade jams, sea buckthorn honey or grated orange peel. You can also use: Sunflower seeds, chopped nuts, garlic, fresh herbs (oregano, basil, dill, parsley, chervil, tarragon, lavender, rosemary, paprika, coriander, turmeric, fenugreek, galangal, parsley, saffron, ginger, pepper, cardamom, chilli and many others. Also seedlings of lentils, mustard and grain.
As salt I use rock salt or sea salt, of course with no iodine additives, fluorine or flow aids. Pepper always comes freshly ground

from the mill, since then the essential oils are most effective. All ingredients are placed in a screw-top jar (300ml) and are shaken vigorously. The amount is usually sufficient for two days and is kept closed in the refrigerator.

Clear salad dressing

4 tbsp lemon juice or fruit vinegar, 6-8 tbsp oil (linseed oil, sunflower oil, walnut oil, olive oil, sesame oil), 1 tsp honey, 1/2 tsp mustard, herbs and spices, fresh or dried, fresh pepper and garlic.

White salad dressing

1 cup of sour cream, 6 tbsp cold-pressed oil (linseed oil, sunflower oil, walnut oil, olive oil, sesame oil), 4 tbsp lemon juice or fruit vinegar, 1/2 tsp mustard, 1 tsp honey, herbs and spices as required, fresh pepper and garlic.

Potato vinaigrette

150g potatoes, cooked until floury, crush with a fork, mix with 100 ml linseed oil; mix 30 g finely chopped shallot, 4 tbsp apple vinegar and 1/2 tsp mustard with 150ml hot vegetable stock. Mix 1 handful of finely chopped herbs (ground elder, parsley, chives, nettles, garlic rocket, oregano, lemon balm, sage, dandelion, etc.) and fresh pepper with all ingredients to form a sauce. Adjust the consistency with vegetable stock. Tastes particularly good with a colourful mixture of leaf salad!

Green salad dressing

1 cup of sour cream, 3 tbsp cold-pressed oil (linseed oil, sunflower oil, walnut oil, olive oil, sesame oil), 3 tbsp lemon juice or fruit vinegar, 1 tsp mustard, 1/2 tsp honey, a bunch of cress or a handful of wild herbs, fresh pepper and garlic. Mix/mash until the sauce turns green.

4.
Warm food

Even the warm food is not heavy. Start with simple dishes. Exchange boiled potatoes for potatoes in skins, pasta for wholemeal pasta and rice for wild rice. Also try millet, spelt or green spelt as side dishes.

Instead of 250 g meat and 150 g vegetables, simply use 250 g vegetables and 150 g meat. Simply omit meat dishes in favour of a vegetable dish every other day or more often. This makes meat special again, and you can spend the money saved at the fishmonger's or organic butcher's for higher quality products. Avoid margarine and inferior, refined frying fats. Replace them with butter and high-quality cold-pressed oils. In the beginning it is better to steam vegetables with a little water and add oil or butter with fresh herbs to the finished cooked vegetables. Otherwise the vital substances are destroyed by heating. In soups, too, butter or oil is added on the plate first. Important: Heated frying fats can limit the tolerance of whole foods!

Stir-fried vegetables

Ingredients: Courgettes, carrots, peppers, parsley root, leek, Brussels sprouts, fennel, pumpkin, onion; everything that the fridge and the season have to offer. Dice at least 3 kinds of vegetables and fry them in some olive oil.

Arrange the vegetable stir-fry on the plate and sprinkle with fresh, chopped tomatoes and herbs. Add some sour cream with garlic or herbs or grated Pecorino cheese.

The vegetable stir-fry can be served alone or with rice, pasta or cooked grain. Alternatively, you can add organic tomato sauce to the vegetables.

Important: Pay attention to the order in which you put the vegetables in the pan. First cabbage, then the vegetables after the required cooking time, using the softer varieties at the end. All vegetables should remain firm to the bite! Finally I like to add raw vegetables to the finished stir-fry (e.g. leek, tomatoes, sprouts).

Roast vegetables

Potatoes, beetroot, paprika, aubergines, cabbage, carrots, beets, asparagus, mushrooms.... Most vegetables can be baked and grilled on a baking tray or grill. Harder vegetables, such as turnips or cabbage, are boiled or blanched for a few minutes to standardise the cooking time.
Clean the vegetables, cut into equal pieces, brush them with a little oil and place the cut surfaces on a greased tray. You can add fresh rosemary, lavender, cumin, garlic, lemon zest or a French herb mixture to the oil. Bake at 175 to 200 degrees for about 20 minutes and serve with garlic sour cream.

Casseroles

500 g thinly sliced firm, boiled potatoes in skins, 1 leek, cut into rings, 1 diced apple, 100 g hard cheese, finely grated, 1 onion, finely diced and sweated until golden, some butter, 1/2 cup vegetable stock, 1/8 litre cream, nutmeg, marjoram or ground cumin, 50 g sunflower seeds.
Spread a casserole dish with butter, layer potatoes and leek, sprinkle with onions, apples and cheese. Mix the stock with some salt, spices and cream and pour over it. Cook at 200 degrees for about 35 minutes. The leek can be replaced with pumpkin, beetroot or black salsify, for example.

Vegetable soups

Potatoes, beetroot, carrots, parsnips, celery, red cabbage, broccoli; almost everything is suitable for a cream or vegetable soup. Clean the vegetables, fry in oil and with onions, fill up with vegetable stock, cook until soft, then purée. Season to taste with herbs and spices and serve with cream or fine oil.

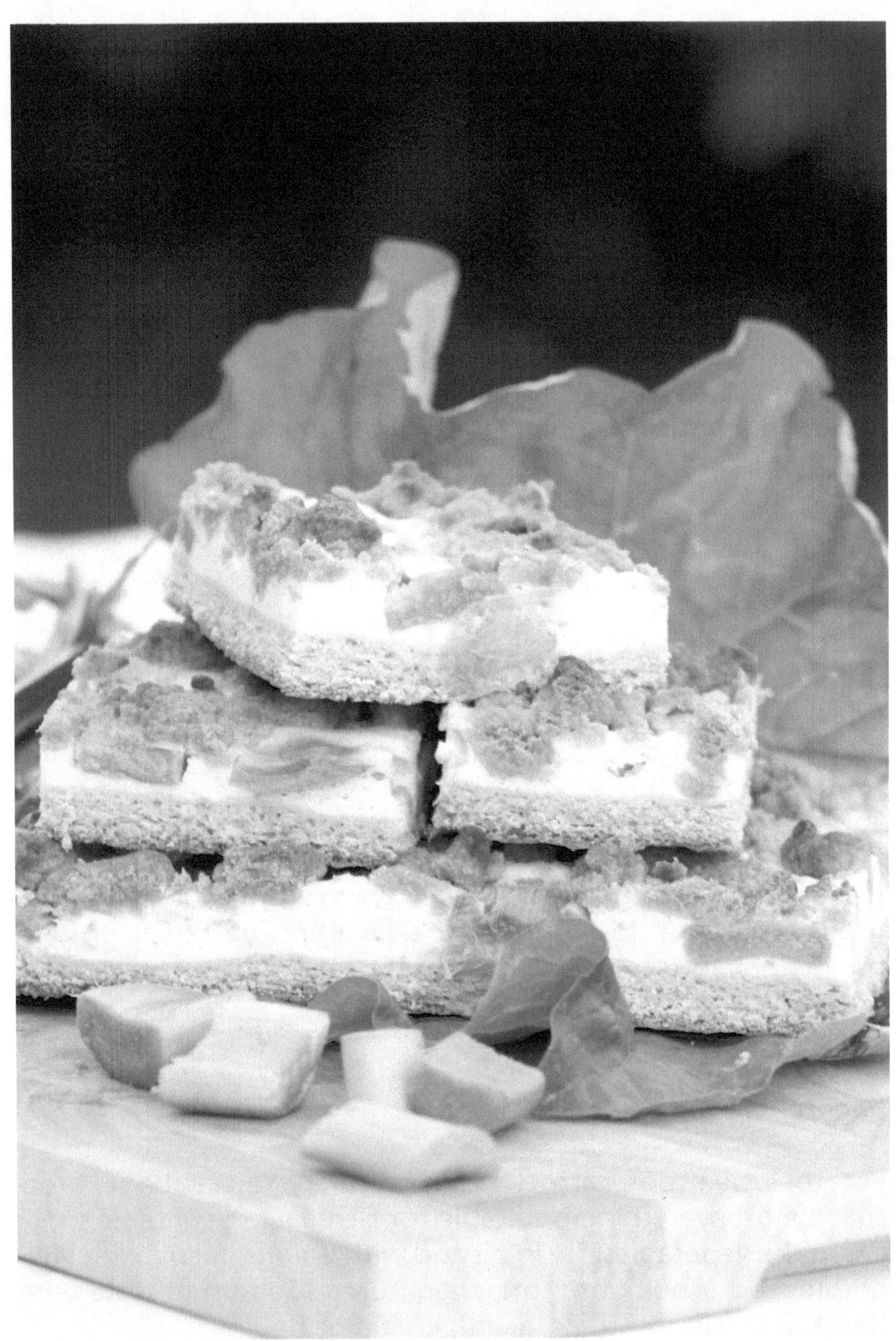

Rhubarb, coconut, quark and crumble pie

Vegetable stock – everything is recycled!

Vegetable waste, peels, stalks, dry parts, i.e. all residues of the vegetable kitchen, are finely chopped and granulated with a chopping knife. I put it all on a tray and let it dry a little. When I have just baked, the tray is sometimes put into the still warm oven to dry. Then I fill everything with some sea salt into a screw-top jar (5:1) and put this jar in the fridge.

When I need vegetable broth, I use a 4-litre saucepan, add about 10 tbsp of the granules and boil it up and let it simmer for an hour on a low heat. Then I pour the broth through a sieve and fill it hot into screw-top jars of various sizes (200-800 ml), close them and keep them in the cellar after they have cooled down. The next soup, sauce or salad dressing is then quicker.

5.

Baking

I bake bread and rolls myself. It tastes good and feels good. I always know what ingredients it contains, and over time, I have gained enough experience to ensure the workload is much less than it was in the beginning!

What is wholemeal bread? Real wholemeal bread is obtained when you put whole grains of grain in the mill, grind them and use this flour for baking. Unfortunately, you will not be able to tell if it is real wholemeal bread based on the colour and texture of the bread.

Wholemeal grains have marginal layers, an oil-containing grain sprout and a starchy flour body. As a result, they are unharmed and therefore can fully germinate. Only grains that can germinate still contain vitamin B1, which is necessary for carbohydrate metabolism, among other things. Ground grain cannot be stored for long because it loses vital substances every day. After about four weeks, almost all vitamins are removed from the flour.

Vegetable pie or pizza

Shortcrust: 500 g spelt or wholemeal emmer flour, 250 g butter, 1 egg, herbal salt or fresh, finely chopped garden herbs.
I prepare a dough from it, roll it into two dough sheets, put it into a food-safe foil bag and put it in the refrigerator for 1 hour. The dough is then put into a tart tin, moulded to the shape and pre-baked in the oven for 10 minutes.

Mix the organic tomato purée with some oil and herbs and then spread on the dough plate. Now I can fill the pie with vegetables of my choice: e.g. grated courgetti or finely chopped pumpkin, grated beetroot, peppers, aubergine, leek, mushrooms, onions, tomatoes; the pie is then baked at 175 degrees for about 35 minutes.
Instead of the tomato paste base, I can also pour over the vegetables: Whisk 2 eggs, 1 cup of sour cream, fresh herbs, nutmeg, salt and pepper and pour over the vegetables, then bake as indicated.

Yeast dough for rolls, bread or cakes

500 g wholemeal wheat or spelt flour, 10 g organic yeast, 10 g sea salt, 40ml sunflower oil, 380ml water, fresh or dried herbs. Dissolve yeast and salt in water. Add the flour and knead well for 10 to 15 minutes. The dough should be soft but not deformed; add water if necessary, cover and leave to rise for 30 minutes in a warm place. Knead again for 5 minutes and let it rise for a further 10 minutes. Roll out the dough into a circle and put it into a greased tin and let it rest again for 5 minutes, then fill the vegetable pie and bake for 20 minutes. The pizza becomes crispier when the base is pre-baked in a hot oven (10 min.), then topped and baked again.
Double the amount and divide the finished dough into two parts. Freeze some for the next pizza.

Spelt rolls

600g wholemeal spelt flour, 350g water, 15g organic yeast, 50ml walnut oil, 12g sea salt, sunflower seeds, linseed or linseed cake as required.
Prepare the dough as above. Form rolls from the dough with wet hands, place on a greased tray and spray with water. Bake in the middle rack for 20 minutes, 10 minutes each at 220 degrees, then at 170 degrees. A bowl of water in the oven provides the necessary moisture – then the baked goods rise better.

6.
Sandwich spreads

Green herb butter

125g butter, various fresh green herbs or wild herbs clean, pluck and chop finely. Add a chopped garlic clove to the butter and mix everything with a blender until the butter is green. Add some sea salt.

Tomato-carrot spread by Ilse Gutjahr

200g organic tomato purée, 2-3 medium-sized carrots, very finely grated, 1 shallot, 125g butter, Provençal herbs: fresh basil, rosemary, thyme, lavender blossoms, oregano, pepper and sea salt. Crush all ingredients and mix to a spreadable mass with a blender

Michaela's fruit spreads

Summer brings us many fruits, such as red, white and black currants, red, yellow and green gooseberries, blueberries, raspber-

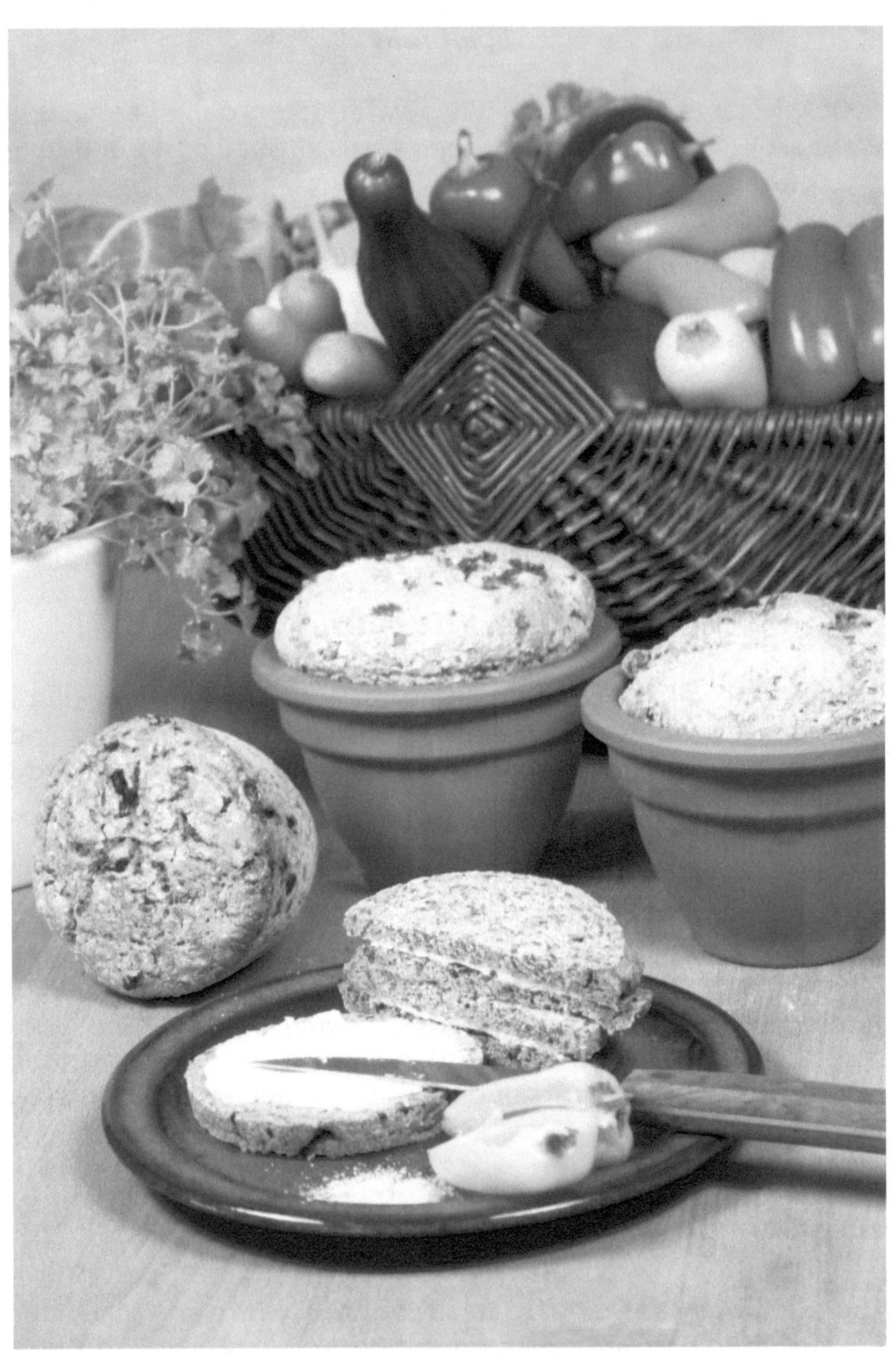

Flowerpot breads with herb and butter

ries and autumn brings aromatic wild fruits. Out of these, I make fruit pulp for the winter and freeze it. The berries are cleaned, puréed and then placed in a sieve to remove the seeds. This fruit pulp is versatile. With a little honey and butter you can make a fruity spread. 2 tablespoons of it mixed in a vinegar/oil salad dressing, results in a fruity salad sauce. Frozen fruit cubes are also great for desserts, lentils or cakes!

7.
Anything is possible
if it tastes good to you

These are just a few suggestions, but you have the cooking ideas graphic, from which you can derive many more recipes: Vegetables can also be used to make wonderful casseroles, röstis or pancakes. With wholemeal dough you can bake with vegetable flat breads, pierogi, filled pasta pockets or vegetable pies.
Sweet, nutritious cakes and tarts are delicious, of course without sugar. And they taste even better! Wholefood cooking offers so many possibilities. Just make a start!

Bon appétit!

Recipes can be found at: www.vitale-landküche.de/recipes

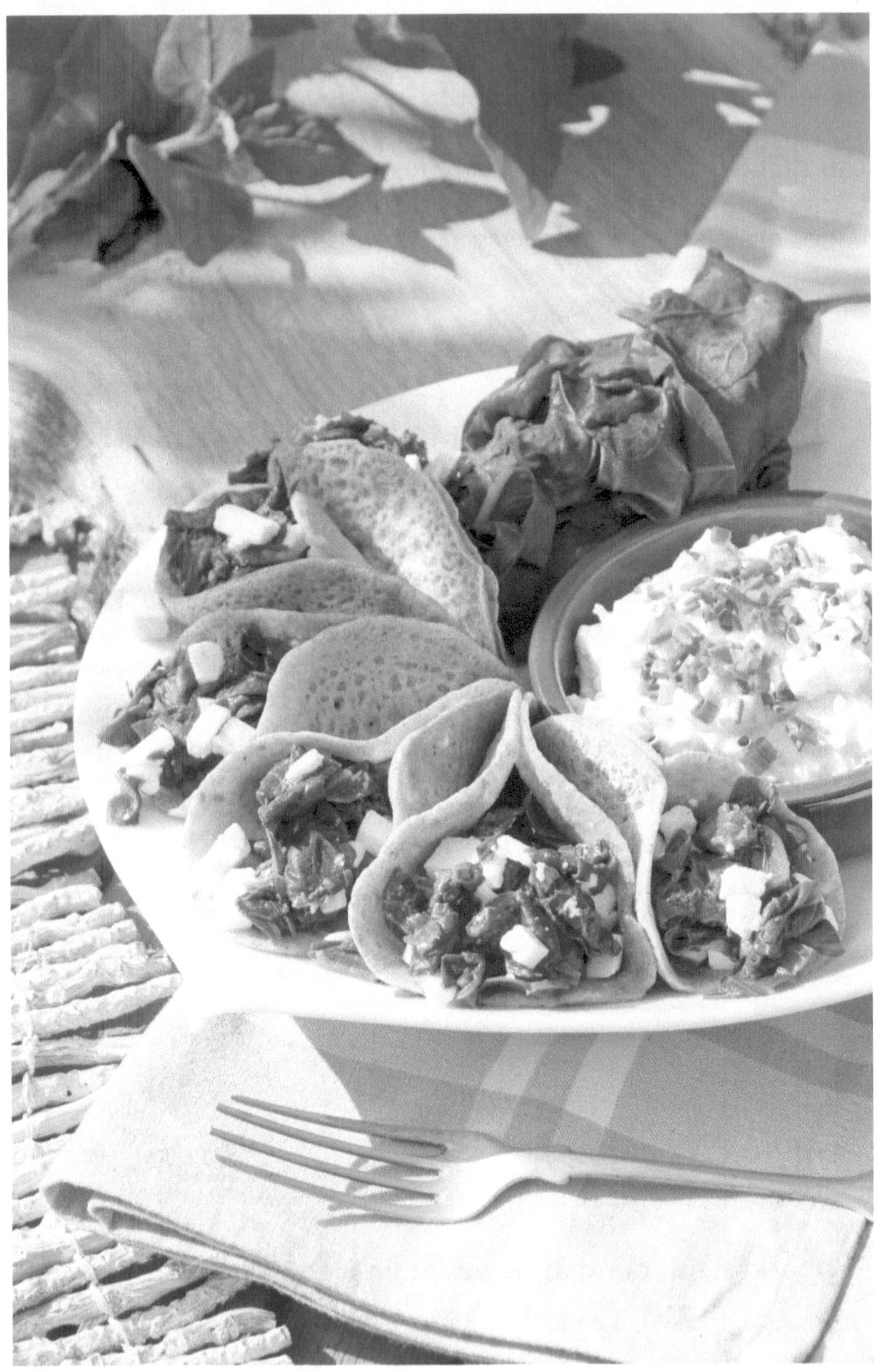

Explanation of terms

Ulcerative colitis

is a chronic inflammatory disease of the large intestine (CID). It is chronic recurrent (intermittent) or chronic continuous. Ulcerative colitis usually starts in the rectum and can spread evenly to the beginning of the small intestine. The division into different forms takes place according to the affected area. The superficial cells of the mucous membrane of the large intestine are affected (not the entire intestinal wall as in Crohn's disease). The mucosa is evenly covered with ulcers. In the initial stage, the inflamed mucous membrane is reddened and bleeds upon contact. Recurring ulcerations lead to gradual destruction of the mucous membrane, whereby the normal folds in the intestinal mucosa are lost.

Gastrointestinal symptoms

The onset is often slow-burning. Prolonged diarrhoea for no apparent reason, recurrent bloody, slimy diarrhoea, persistent abdominal pain in the left lower abdomen, sometimes massive intestinal bleeding and colic, the complete inability to hold the stool.

General symptoms

The signs of the disease are usually not limited to the abdominal and intestinal area. They are usually associated with a general feeling of being unwell. Fever, fatigue, loss of performance, exhaustion, loss of appetite and weight, anaemia, arthritis, skin changes, eye infections, dry mucous membranes, symptoms of nutrient deficiency, food intolerances, growth disorders in children.

References

Unsere Nahrung – unser Schicksal
[Our Diet – Our Fate]
Dr. med. Max Otto Bruker, emu Verlag

Leber-, Galle-, Magen-, Darm- und Bauchspeicheldrüsenerkrankungen Ernährungsbehandlung mit vitalstoffreicher Vollwertkost
[Liver, Gallbladder, gastrointestinal and pancreatic diseases – Nutritional treatment with nutritious whole foods]
Dr. med. Max Otto Bruker, emu Verlag

Zucker Zucker, Krank durch Fabrikzucker
[Sugar, Sugar, Sick due to Refined Sugars]
Dr. med. Max Otto Bruker, Ilse Gutjahr, emu Verlag

Lebensbedingte Krankheiten
[Lifestyle-related diseases
Everyone experiences life crises, worry and stress today]
This book describes how you can successfully meet these challenges in life.
Dr. med. Max Otto Bruker, emu Verlag

Seele – Sucht – Sehnsucht, Wege zur Klarheit
[Soul – Addiction – Longing, Ways to Clarity]
Dr. phil. Mathias Jung, emu Verlag

Mein Charakter – mein Schicksal
[My Character – My Fate]
Dr. phil. Mathias Jung, emu Verlag

Die Suppe lügt [The Soup Lies]
Hans-Ulrich Grimm, Knaur, 1999

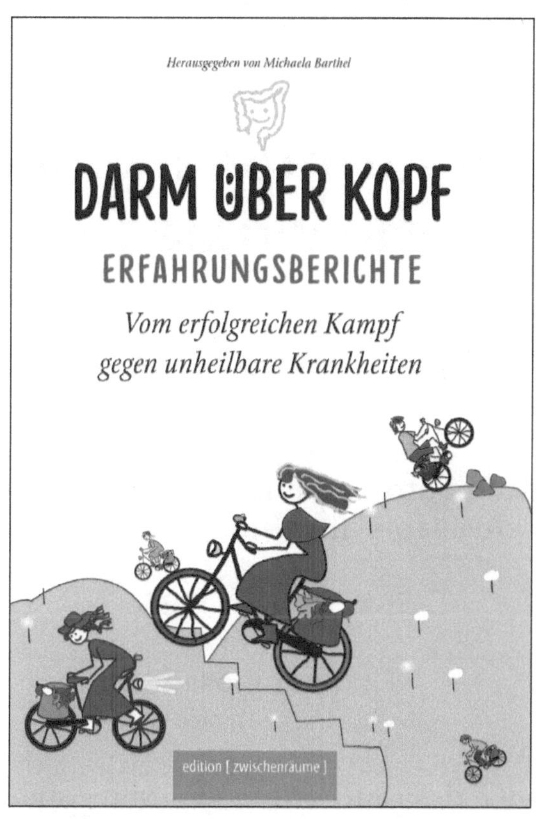

Go with your Gut Instinct

TESTIMONIALS
The successful fight against incurable diseases

Published by Michaela Barthel
ISBN 978-3-9815286-4-0

Find out more from: www.vitale-landküche.de

Every person has just ONE life. The author has been given a second life!
Thirteen stories from "incurably-ill" patients, who have taken up the fight
against their illness – and who are now on the winning side. What have
the main players changed in their lives? Nothing that you can't do too ...

A nutritional guide
for the whole family

Excellent ideas, lots of tips & tasty recipes

A book by Michaela Barthel
with lots of photos, graphs, tables and detailed recipes
Available at the beginning of 2017

ISBN 978-3-9815286-3-3

Find out more from:
www.vitale-landküche.de

We all have a desire for lifelong vitality and health. It has often been recognised that nutrition plays a crucial role in this. The road to a change in diet is paved with questions such as: Is wholefood a diet? Does it involve a lot of work? How do I change to a wholefood diet? Will I feel full?
Is it expensive? But I don't tolerate very much! How can I persuade my family, my children to get involved? These and similar questions have been asked again and again during lectures, courses and consultations over the last four years. They have prompted me to publish this guide to the basics of wholefood cuisine with many practical tips and recipes.

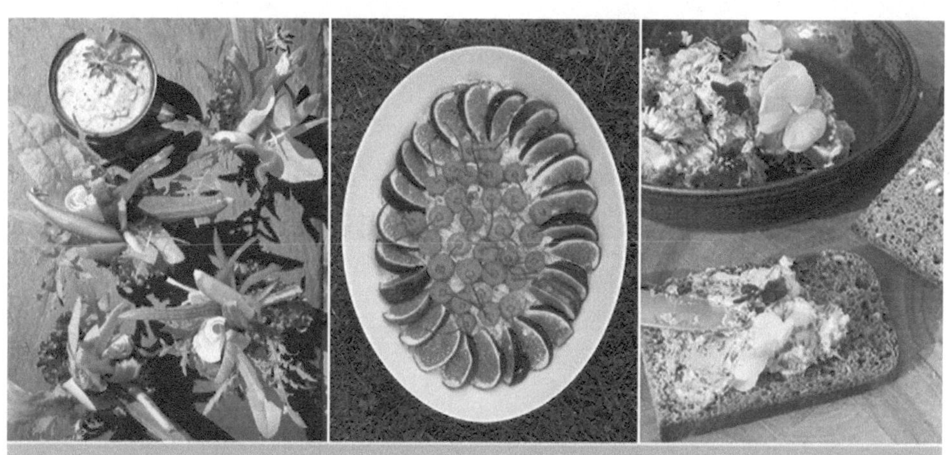

Eine Vollwert-Fibel für die ganze Familie

Gute Tipps, einfache Tricks & leckere Rezepte

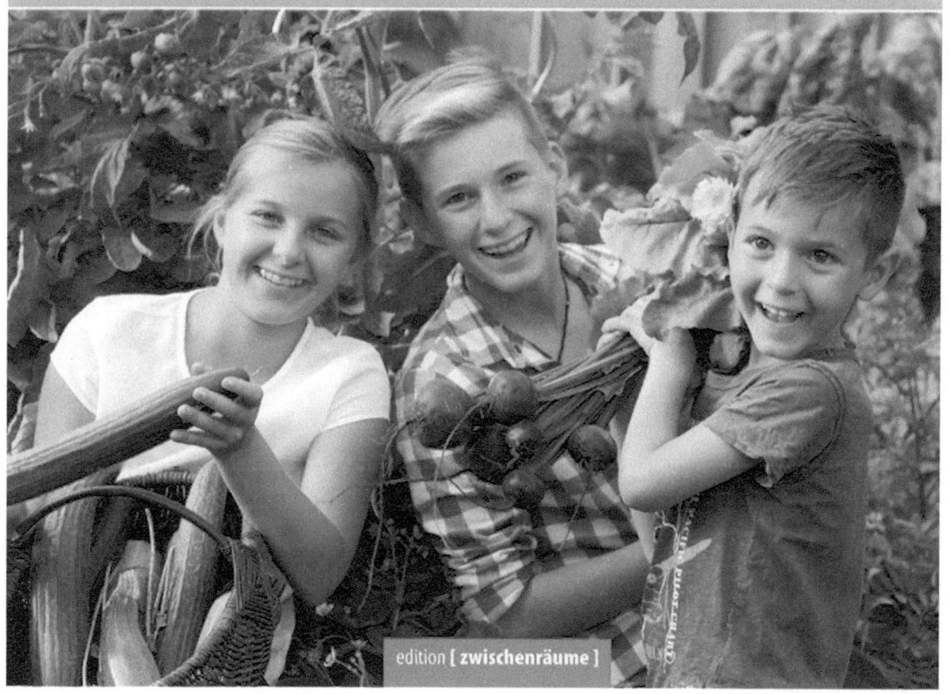

contents